THE
STEVIA
COOKBOOK

THE STEVIA COOKBOOK

RAY SAHELIAN, MD
DONNA GATES

AVERY
a member of Penguin Putnam Inc.

Cover Designer: Doug Brooks
Typesetter: Gary Rosenberg
In-House Editor: Marie Caratozzolo

Avery
a member of
Penguin Putnam Inc.
375 Hudson Street
New York, NY 10014
www.penguinputnam.com

Cataloging-in-Publication Data

Sahelian, Ray.
 The stevia cookbook : cooking with nature's calorie-free sweetener /
Ray Sahelian & Donna Gates.
   p. cm.
 Includes bibliographical references and index.
 ISBN 0–89529–926–7
 1. Cookery (stevia). 2. Stevia rebaudiana. I. Gates, Donna. II. Title.
TX819.S75S24   1999
641.5'63—dc21   99–11740
                                                  CIP

Printed in the United States of America

20 19 18 17 16 15 14

Contents

Actions taken today affect our children for generations to come . . . therefore, this book is dedicated:

To those extraordinary individuals within the health food industry who work tirelessly in their respective organizations and businesses to bring the truth to the American public.

And to those enlightened, young American chefs who, responding to an inner calling, know that they have a key role to play in helping our country become healthy.

And to our young adults and our children who, unaware of their roles as of yet, will be waking up and remembering that creating a healthy body and a balanced mind is critical in order to fulfill their spiritual mission of creating a happier, healthier world.

Acknowledgments

I sincerely wish to thank Linda and Bill Bonvie, a New Jersey-based sister-brother writing team for researching much of the information relating to the FDA ruling on stevia. They first published this story in the January/February 1996 issue of *New Age Journal*, and later coauthored *The Stevia Story* with Donna Gates.

Meeting with Donna Gates was a fortuitous event that gave rise to the eventual publication of this book. From the very start, I was impressed with Donna's genuine motivation to spread the good news about stevia.

The patient guidance and support from project editor Marie Caratozzolo and publisher Rudy Shur are also greatly appreciated.

Last but not least, I am grateful to my mother, Jackie, for spending long hours kitchen-testing the recipes.

—Ray Sahelian

Years ago, when I first discovered stevia, no recipes existed that could guide us in eliminating sugar from our favorite foods and replacing it with this simple, sweet-tasting herb. Even in other countries where stevia had been in use for decades or even centuries, no cookbook like this one had ever been written. So, along with Dr. Ray Sahelian, I took on the challenge of creating one. It was a frustrating journey—one with lots of mistakes and wasted ingredients. The gods must have been looking down on me, however, and John Wright walked into my life. Together, we created the recipes in this book. For him, the pie recipes, as well as the sauces and entrées came easily. So I am deeply grateful for his creative and joyful presence in my life. Thank you, John. It is much more fun to fight a battle with someone like you beside me.

I am grateful, too, for my coauthor, Ray Sahelian, especially for his attention to detail and his wonderful sense of humor. And a special thank you to Ray's mom, Jackie Sahelian, for testing the recipes so quickly and making valuable comments and suggestions. Marie Caratozzolo from Avery Publishing deserves a medal of honor for her patience with me. And so does Rudy Shur, president of Avery, for believing, like Ray and I do, that after this publication, stevia will become a household word.

—Donna Gates

Preface

What if there were an all-natural sweetener that:

- was 200 to 300 times sweeter than regular sugar?

- had no calories?

- was suitable for diabetics?

- was safe for children?

- did not cause cavities?

- was heat stable and, therefore, could be used for cooking and baking?

- was a great alternative to synthetic sweeteners?

- was easily blended with other sweeteners, such as honey?

- was already widely and safely consumed in many countries around the world for decades?

Wouldn't you expect that you would have heard about such a product? And wouldn't you figure that many of our sweetened foods would contain it instead of sugar or artificial chemical-based sweeteners?

Well, there *is* such a remarkable no-calorie sweetener. It is called stevia and is derived from a plant of the daisy family that grows in South America. Just beginning to get noticed in the United States, stevia is slowly becoming one of the most popular and widely used sweeteners in the world.

This book tells the story of stevia—from its use by South American Indian tribes for hundreds of years to its more recent popularity in Japan for nearly two decades. Through documented studies, as well as the track records of those who have used stevia for many years, you will learn about the safety of this product, which is bound to revolutionize the way we think about sugar. And, with over 100 taste-tempting recipes and variations presented for your enjoyment, you will learn how to use stevia as a natural sweetener in a wide variety of foods and beverages.

Introduction

"What would you like to drink?" asked the waiter.

I flipped the menu over to examine the choices listed on the back. The options were herbal teas, vegetable juices, and fruit juices. I was about to ask what kind of herbal teas they had when I was interrupted.

"Bring him a glass of water with lemon on the side," said Donna, the woman sitting across from me.

I was taken aback a little by her assertiveness. We were at Inaka, a natural food restaurant in Los Angeles. This was my first meeting with Donna, who had been introduced to me by a mutual friend. Donna is a nutritionist who lives in Atlanta, Georgia, but was in Los Angeles visiting her daughter.

"I want you to try a natural sweetener called stevia," she added.

I had heard a little about stevia (pronounced stēē′•vi•a) a year earlier. It had been touted as a natural alternative to both table sugar and the synthetic sweeteners currently being marketed. At the time, I hadn't paid much attention to these claims because I couldn't imagine a natural sweetener as powerful as an artificial one like saccharin or aspartame. At the most, I figured it had perhaps similar sweetening potential as honey.

The waiter brought the glass of water and placed it on the table. Next to it he put a small plate with two lemon wedges.

"Now, squeeze the lemon in the water," instructed Donna.

I followed her instructions and squeezed the lemon into the glass, first making sure I removed the seeds with a fork.

"Now add five drops of this stevia liquid extract," she added, as she handed me a small dropper-style bottle filled with the clear liquid.

Before I added the drops, I took a sip from the glass. The water had a definite lemon flavor. After adding the drops, I watched them make their way to the bottom of the glass, partially dissolving along the way. I quickly took a sip. Frankly, I was disappointed. Just as I had suspected, it wasn't very sweet. Being familiar with synthetic sweeteners, I knew a natural substance couldn't compete. The claims about stevia were obviously hyped.

"Did you stir it?" asked Donna.

I hadn't. With a spoon, I swirled the water around a few times, then I took another sip—I couldn't believe it!

"Wow, it tastes as sweet as if I had put a couple teaspoons of sugar in the glass," I said excitedly. I took another sip. "This just may be my imagination, Donna, but even the lemon flavor seems more enhanced."

"Yes, it does bring out the flavor of lemons, as well as a number of other foods," she informed me.

"Where do you buy this stuff?"

"Most health food stores carry stevia. With time, I believe it will become available in grocery and other retail stores. I carry a small bottle of it in its liquid form with me at all times."

"What about calories?" I asked, trying to figure out what was wrong with stevia.

"None," was Donna's reply. She continued, "In my opinion, stevia is the ideal no-calorie sweetener. It comes from a plant that grows in South America, where the leaves have been used as a sweetener for hundreds of years. In the early 1970s, the Japanese learned of stevia and they have been using it in soy products, soft drinks, and a number of other foods. Unfortunately, the American general public knows little about it."

"Why is that?" I wondered aloud.

"In 1991, the FDA banned the import of stevia to the United States as a sweetener; however, in 1995, it allowed stevia to become available again as a dietary supplement. I've done extensive reviews of the research on stevia, and tests have shown it to be very safe." She continued, "I have been using stevia instead of sugar for a number of years and have created a number of great tasting stevia recipes."

When I had finished my drink, I asked for another glass of water. I squeezed the second piece of lemon into the glass. This time, I added only four drops of stevia. The drink was still sweet and delicious—as good as sugared lemonade. When the second glass was empty, the waiter filled it again and gave me another dish of lemon wedges. This time I added three drops, which was still adequate for sweetening the lemonade.

Toward the end of my very enjoyable dinner with Donna, I became more and more convinced that there was something special about stevia. I wanted to find out everything I could about it—exactly what it is, how it works, and what, if any, side effects it has on the body. I was determined to fully investigate the scientific studies published on stevia and learn more about the FDA's motivation in banning its import as a sweetener in 1991. Most important, I was determined to discover if stevia is safe for long-term human consumption.

I took the last sip from my glass and said, "I can't believe so little is known in this country about a natural sweetener that works so well. If stevia is everything you say it is, sooner or later it will be big news. It could be used extensively as a replacement for sugar and artificial sweeteners.

Donna agreed.

I remarked to Donna that the manufacturers of artificial sweeteners were likely to feel threatened by this safe, natural alternative for their patented products. She concurred that they could be shedding some sweet tears over it.

My mind went into overdrive as it raced with ideas. "I'm guessing that diabetics would certainly be able to take advantage of stevia."

"That's right," Donna replied.

"For children, or anyone for that matter, it would be a safe alternative for high-calorie, sugar-sweetened drinks and snacks that are so popular."

Donna continued, "And don't forget about those people who are trying to lose weight but find it difficult to break from their sugar addiction, or those who are concerned with the potential risks of artificial sweeteners."

"What about stevia's role in tooth decay?" I asked.

"At least one study has shown that stevia does not cause dental cavities. This means it can be used to naturally sweeten candy, chewing gum, mouthwash, and even toothpaste."

I looked at Donna. There was little doubt in my mind that she genuinely believed in the potential benefits of stevia as an excellent alternative to currently available sweeteners.

"Donna, I have a proposal for you," I said.

"What's that?"

"How would you like to spread the stevia story with me?"

"Absolutely," she responded.

At that very moment, we joined forces and began to discuss our mission—our goal was to gather as much information about stevia as we could, then share our findings with the world. We researched, analyzed studies, and even kitchen-tested stevia in a number of recipes. As the result of our efforts, we have written *The Stevia Cookbook.* In it you will learn all about stevia—what it is, its many forms, and the number of ways it can be used. You'll learn about the FDA ban on its import as a sweetener in 1991, and the lifting of that ban in 1995, allowing it to be distributed as a dietary supplement. Most important, you'll learn of the safety of stevia as seen through animal and human studies, as well as through its long-time use in Japan and in South America. As a final bonus, over 100 taste-tempting stevia recipes and variations are presented. These include hearty breakfast fare such as pancakes and waffles (complete with stevia-sweetened homemade syrup), naturally sweetened beverages like refreshing ginger ale and hot cocoa, and a wealth of luscious cakes, cookies, puddings, and other assorted sweet treats.

After reading *The Stevia Cookbook,* we know you will be as amazed as we are with stevia's impressive qualities. We're sure you will find it easy to incorporate as a natural sweetener in your life.

PART ONE

THE STORY OF STEVIA

CHAPTER 1

Donna's Story— Dealings With the FDA

Many years ago, I became interested in developing and promoting a more natural lifestyle. I learned that each of us has an internal ecosystem that must be cared for if we are to achieve and maintain optimal health. This healthier way of life involved, among other things, incorporating whole foods into my diet. Early on, however, it became clear that I was missing one of the key ingredients of this diet—a healthy sugar substitute. Uncomfortable with artificial sweeteners such as aspartame and saccharin, I began the search for a safe natural alternative.

STEVIA—THE NO-CALORIE MIRACLE

I first heard about stevia in 1990 from a marketing firm that was promoting it as the component of a facemask. The edible green-colored stevia syrup (derived from stevia leaves) was packaged along with a small bottle of clay. The instructions recommended that the clay be blended with the stevia syrup and applied to the face. But it was the syrup's potential as a sweetener that interested me. I tried it. It was intensely sweet with a licorice-like aftertaste. Later I learned that I had taken far too much, a common mistake made by first-time users. Fortunately, a much more flavorful version of stevia came my way.

The Envelope With the White Powder

While I presently live in Atlanta, Georgia, in 1990 I was living in Washington, D.C. One night, while having dinner with two friends who worked at the Chinese Embassy, I mentioned my frustration in finding an adequate sugar substitute. Several weeks later, to my surprise, my friends presented me with an envelope containing a white powder. It was a sample of stevioside crystals (a sweet substance derived from the stevia plant). The crystals had come from Chinese-grown stevia plants and had been extracted through an award-winning procedure that had been developed in Japan. Through this process, the stevia plant's super-sweet elements are extracted, leaving behind the plant's licorice-tasting residue. This concentrated powder, by weight, is 200 to 300 times sweeter than sugar.

I was thrilled! Here was a widely used, totally natural sweetener that had virtually no calories. I immediately began experimenting with it—baking with it, adding it to beverages, and making stevia-sweetened desserts. I soon began sharing my stevia and stevia-sweetened recipes with friends and family, as well as my students and clients. They, too, began to use stevia in place of sugar and were amazed by its sweet taste. Soon thereafter, I arranged for delivery of a large amount of stevia to be sent to me from China.

FDA RULING SOURS THE SWEET STEVIA STORY

In 1991, a curious thing happened. The Food and Drug Administration (FDA) labeled stevia an "unsafe food additive" and issued an alert that blocked the importation of stevia into the United States. This seemed to be a really peculiar development. After all, so few people knew about stevia, and only a few health food stores carried it. As the months rolled by, I noticed that the health food stores, knowing of the ban, continued to sell stevia quite openly. It moved quickly off the shelves as loyal customers bought the last available supplies. Then it was gone.

During this time, I did an enormous amount of research. First, I used the Freedom of Information Act request to obtain all of the information on stevia that was then in the hands of the FDA. Nowhere in the literature was there any indication of stevia causing ill effects in humans. Plus, I was using stevia regularly, as were many people I knew. No one had experienced any adverse effects. Everyone loved it.

In 1992, I moved to Atlanta. By then, the FDA had succeeded in stonewalling the marketing of stevia by refusing to consider petitions that sought to have it officially placed on the GRAS (generally recognized as safe) list. This list includes herbs and nutrients that have had a history of safe use. I found it odd that the FDA refused to add stevia to the list, considering animal studies had indicated saccharin to be potentially cancer causing, yet it was being widely sold. In fact, the SWEET 'N LOW package clearly mentions this concern. Why was saccharin readily available, yet stevia—a natural sweetener used for centuries in South America—not? I decided to take a stand.

The ban on stevia put its supporters in a classic "Catch-22" position. In order to prove that stevia is safe for human consumption as a food additive, millions of dollars (and years of effort) would be required to move this herb through the FDA approval process. However, those who invest all of this money would not be able to recoup their investment since they would not be able to patent stevia. Any number of manufacturers could import stevia and begin marketing it. This is because, unlike aspartame and saccharin, stevia is an herb and not a synthetic creation by a pharmaceutical company. Economists call this a "free rider"—one person or company bears the expense of obtaining the approval, and then everyone else is able to take a free ride in marketing the product.

SWEET REVENGE—THE DIETARY SUPPLEMENT HEALTH AND EDUCATION ACT

During 1993, the FDA miscalculated. It attempted to take control of dietary supplements and herbal products by limiting their availability to the public. To everyone's surprise, a massive grassroots movement objected to this intrusion into a person's right to self-medicate with dietary supplements. Various natural food industry groups organized to respond to this threat, and a few senators and members of Congress rallied behind them. Senator Orrin Hatch from Utah was instrumental in solidifying the movement's opposition. Ads began appearing everywhere, even on television. I remember seeing one advertisement of a consumer in his kitchen opening a bottle of vitamin C. Just as he was about to pop one of the vitamins in his mouth, FDA agents burst through the door, handcuffed him, and dragged him out of his house for prosecution. Of course, this was quite an exaggeration, but it made the point. The public rallied, afraid to have its multivitamins taken away.

Based on continued pressure from the public, the natural foods industry, and the American Herbal Products Association, Congress passed the Dietary Supplement Health and Education Act in the fall of 1994. This law eased restrictions on a number of dietary supplements for sale to the public. The FDA could no longer classify supplements as food additives. This meant that dietary supplements did not have to be subjected to intensive safety testing before their introduction to the American consumer. You may recall that the hormone melatonin became available to the public as a consequence of this law. And, as a result of a vitamin company notifying the FDA of its intention to market stevia, the FDA lifted its ban in 1995.

STEVIA CITIZENSHIP REINSTATED—WILL THE SUGAR INDUSTRY NOW HOBBLE ON CANE?

So stevia began to flow back into the United States. Not as a sweetener, mind you, but as a dietary supplement. Its natural sweetening qualities, the FDA warned, would still be considered a "technical effect," and, therefore, should not be mentioned. While the natural foods industry was encouraged by the lifting of the import ban, few had wanted to attract the attention of the FDA by including stevia in their products and advertising it for what it actually is—a sweetener. Because stevia remains in legal limbo, food manufacturers are apprehensive about using it in their products.

SOME FINAL WORDS

I know all of this must sound difficult to believe, yet it's true. As this book goes to press, a natural, no-calorie, safe-for-diabetics, non-pharmaceutical sweetener that is already widely used in other countries, including Japan (whose Ministry of Health is notoriously stricter than the FDA), cannot be openly sold as a sweetener in this country.

I've always wondered whether the FDA was pressured by the sugar industry or manufacturers of artificial sweeteners to ban the importation of stevia. After all, if stevia can be imported and sold by anyone, it could be a major economic threat to these companies.

CHAPTER 2

The Super Sweetener

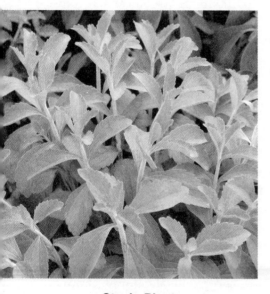

Stevia Plant

Known by the official taxonomy name of *Stevia rebaudiana*, stevia is a plant of the daisy family that grows naturally in South America. At its full maturity, the plant reaches a height of close to three feet, and its green leaves contain large amounts (up to 5 percent dry weight) of stevioside—a sweetener estimated to be 300 times as sweet as table sugar (Isima, 1976).

At least 150 species of stevia are believed to exist in North and South America. In a 1982 study, more than 110 species of stevia were tested for their sweetness. *Stevia rebaudiana* was found to be the sweetest, although 18 other species were found to exhibit a sweet taste as well (Soejarto, 1982). It's quite possible that there are other untested stevia species that are as sweet as *Stevia rebaudiana*.

The researchers in the above study made an interesting observation. They found fragments of a sixty-two-year-old *Stevia rebaudiana* leaf that exhibited potent sweetness. This is significant because it indicates that the chemicals within the herb are very stable and have the ability to withstand time.

CHARACTERISTICS OF STEVIA

Stevia, of course, is very sweet, and it has only a minimal aftertaste. A human study done in 1977 indicates that the quality of stevia's sweetness is preferable to that of aspartame or saccharin (Abe, 1977).

One study conducted in Japan in 1976 concluded that pure stevia extract was 300 times as sweet as sucrose (or table sugar) at 0.4 percent sucrose concentration. It was 100 times sweeter when compared to a 10 percent concentration.

There are normally hundreds of chemicals present within any herbal product or extract. It's sometimes very difficult to identify every single component of an herb. Resistant to heat and time, the compounds within stevia are very stable and can last for decades. Preliminary studies with stevia have shown that it contains certain chemicals, including stevioside and rebaudioside, that provide a sweet taste (Kinghorn, 1984). As mentioned earlier, stevioside makes up about 5 percent of the leaves' dry weight, while rebaudioside makes up 2 percent. Found at a lower concentration than stevioside, rebaudioside is a more pleasant-tasting sweet substance (Crammer, 1987).

Additionally, the oily part of stevia contains a number of sterols including stigmasterol, beta-sitosterol, and campesterol (D'Agostino, 1984). Stevioside is a diterpenic carboxylic alcohol with three glucose molecules $C_{38}H_{60}O_{18}$ (Mosettig, 1955).

GOD'S GIFT TO THE GUARANI

Certain Indian tribes in South America have used stevia for hundreds of years, possibly even before Columbus landed there (Lee, 1979). Since the natural habitat of this plant is northeastern Paraguay near the Brazilian border, the Indians of that region, named the Guarani, were the first to take advantage of its sweet properties. They called it *kaa he-e,* a native term that translates as "sweet herb." The Guarani were aware that the leaves of the wild stevia shrub had a sweetening power unlike anything else, and they commonly used the leaves to enhance the taste of bitter maté, a tea-like beverage. Stevia leaves were chewed for their sweet taste, and added to medicinal potions, as well.

The widespread native use of stevia was chronicled by the Spaniards in historical documents preserved in the Paraguayan National Archives in Asunción, Paraguay. As settlers moved into the region, they learned of this shrub and started using it. By the 1800s, daily stevia consumption had become well entrenched throughout Paraguay and in the neighboring countries of Brazil and Argentina.

Credit for the discovery of stevia by a Westerner goes to an Italian botanist named Moises Santiago Bertoni. He first learned of what he described as, "this very strange plant" from Indian guides while exploring Paraguay's eastern forests in 1887. It was twelve years later when he was presented with a packet of stevia fragments and broken leaves, which he received from a friend who had gotten them from maté plantations.

Bertoni named this variety of stevia *rebaudiana* in honor of a Paraguayan chemist named Rebaudi, who subsequently became the first to extract the plant's sweet constituent. (As mentioned earlier, one of the chemicals responsible for stevia's sweetness is rebaudioside, also named after Rebaudi). Bertoni was quite excited about his discovery. "In placing in the mouth the smallest particle of any portion of the leaf or twig," he wrote, "one is surprised at the strange and extreme sweetness contained therein. A fragment of the leaf only a few millimeters in size suffices to keep the mouth sweet for an hour; a few small leaves are sufficient to sweeten a strong cup of coffee or tea."

In 1903 Bertoni began his full study of this plant. In 1905, he published his results and assigned this plant to the genus *Stevia.*

CULTIVATION AND GROWING PAINS

Bertoni's "discovery" led to his identifying, analyzing, and naming this plant. In addition, his work was a turning point for stevia in another very real sense: Prior to 1900, the stevia plant had grown only in the wild, with consumption limited to those with access to its natural habitat. After Bertoni's studies, stevia became ripe for cultivation. In 1908, a ton of dried leaves was harvested—the very first stevia crop. Before long, stevia plantations began springing up throughout South America. Ironically, this development corresponded with a marked reduction in the plant's natural growth area. This reduction was due in part to the clearing of forests by timber interests and, to an extent, the removal of thousands of stevia plants for transplantation (Soejarto, 1983). Transplantation was necessary because growing stevia from seed is very difficult. Consequently, its use began to increase dramatically, both in and beyond Latin America.

As word of this unique herb began to spread, so too did interest in its potential as a marketable commodity. Stevia was first brought to the attention of the United States government in 1918 by a botanist for the Department of Agriculture (USDA). He had learned about the "remarkable sweetness" of stevia while drinking maté.

Stevia was presented to the USDA in 1921 by American Trade Commissioner George Brady as a "new sugar plant with great commercial possibilities." Brady took note of stevia's nontoxicity and its ability to be used in its natural state, with only drying and grinding required. He also conveyed the claims that it was "an ideal and safe sugar for diabetics." In a memo to the Latin American Division of the USDA, Brady further stated that he was "desirous of seeing it placed before any American companies liable to be interested, as it is very probable that it will be of great commercial importance."

A SWEET REDISCOVERY—SAYONARA SACCHARIN

While nothing came of stevia's early show of interest in the United States, an event occurred in France in 1931 that would later prove significant. Two chemists isolated the most prevalent of several compounds that gives the stevia leaf its sweet taste, a pure white crystalline extract they named stevioside (Bridel, 1931). One United

States government researcher, Dr. Hewitt Fletcher, described this extract as "the sweetest natural product yet found." Unfortunately, he then added, "It is natural to ask, 'of what use is stevioside?' The answer at this point is 'none.'" The Japanese, however, did not take this researcher's opinion too seriously.

Consistent with a popular movement in the 1960s to deter the use of chemicals in the food supply, the Japanese government partially restricted the use of artificial sweeteners. Originally introduced to Japan in the mid 1970s by a consortium of food-product manufacturers, stevioside and other stevia products quickly caught on. By 1988, these products reportedly represented approximately 41 percent of the market share of potently sweet substances consumed in Japan (Kinghorn, 1992). In addition to widespread use as a table-top sweetener, stevia is also used by the Japanese to sweeten a variety of food products, including ice cream, bread, candies, pickles, seafood, vegetables, and soft drinks. It is even added to chewing gum.

Japan's experience proved several other significant facts about this phenomenal plant, including its safety and adaptability. Stevia is able to be grown throughout most of Japan's temperate islands, albeit under special hothouse conditions.

STEVIA GOES GLOBAL

The spread of stevia has not been limited to Japan. Today it is also grown and used in a number of other countries throughout the world. By the mid 1980s, stevia's reputation and potential commercial value had finally sparked the interest of various companies in the United States. Celestial Seasonings, for instance, began using crushed, powdered stevia leaves to create herbal teas that were sweet yet noncaloric. No side effects were reported. With the addition of stevia to a number of popular brands of herbal tea (as a sweetener and flavor enhancer), this remarkable ancient sweet herb of the Guarani Indians was at last poised to make a delayed debut in the American marketplace.

By this time, however, powerful market forces were at work. A major artificial sweetener industry began to notice the potential threat of stevia—a sweetener that was natural, calorie-free, and safe; one that could be cultivated and sold by anyone. Once stevia had been introduced to the herbal scene in the United States and began growing in market share, the FDA launched an aggressive campaign to nip it in the bud. In 1987, the FDA began notifying companies selling herbal products that they could no longer market stevia because it was not an approved food additive.

THE FDA VERSUS FORTY BOXES OF THAT SOUTH AMERICAN WHITE POWDER

Yes, your federal agents are hard at work, protecting you from the dangers of white powders imported from South America. However, this particular white powder is not snorted, it's added to your breakfast tea or your lemonade.

Linda Bonvie and Bill Bonvie, a brother and sister writing team, published an excellent article in the January/February 1996 issue of *New Age Journal*. In it, they investigated the possible behind-the-scenes motivation of the FDA's import ban.

The article begins with the big-time "drug bust" that occurred in Texas shortly after the stevia import ban took effect. The so-called "bust:"

> . . . took place on a summer day in 1991, when a bevy of armed federal marshals raided the Arlington, Texas, warehouse of businessman Oscar Rodes. There, they served him with a warrant and proceeded to seize his most recent stevia shipment. "They didn't give me any advance notice or anything," Rodes recalls. "They came in my office in the warehouse, and that's when they showed me the papers and took everything away."
>
> Rodes himself was not taken into custody. The arrest warrant was for the boxes he had just imported from South America that contained dried stevia leaves and a white powder extracted from them. "They just asked me to open the warehouse door, and they backed up the truck and loaded it up," he recalls. "They said they were going to burn it. I was surprised—all the marshals, ready to go and take away my teas."

A search on the internet at the FDA website (www.fda.org) reveals the following alert, which was posted on December 19, 1995 to guide FDA agents in the field:

Subject:

Automatic detention of stevia leaves, extract of stevia leaves, and foods containing stevia, unless explicitly labeled as a dietary supplement.

Problem:

Unsafe food additive.

Reason for Alert:

Stevioside, the extract of stevia, has reportedly been approved for use in foods in Brazil and Japan. The product is used in these countries as a table top sweetener in virtually all food commodities and as a flavor enhancer in such products as teas.

With regard to its use in foods, stevia is not an approved food additive nor is it affirmed as GRAS (generally recognized as safe) in the United States. Available toxicological information on stevia is inadequate to demonstrate its safety as a food additive. However, with regard to its use in dietary supplements, stevia is not subject to food additive regulations.

Stevia leaves and stevioside have been offered for entry both in bulk and in finished products. Examples of products detained because of stevia include teas, drinks, seafood, fruits, vegetables, and candies.

Guidance:

Districts may detain without physical examination all products identified on the attachment to this alert. If review of the labeling or import paper-work reveals stevia leaves, stevioside, or products containing stevioside, districts may detain these items without physical examination, unless explicitly labeled as a dietary supplement, or for use solely as a dietary ingredient in the manufacture of a dietary supplement product. For questions or issues concerning science, policy, sample collection, or analysis, contact the FDA, Division of Field Science at 301–443–3320. For the full report, see website www.fda.gov//ora/fiars/ora_import_ia4506.html.

SWEETENING THE PALM?

Just what prompted the FDA to intervene forcefully in the market-ing of stevia is difficult to fully unravel. Rumors persist that the catalyst was a "trade complaint" from a company that did not want stevia made available to consumers. As of this writing, no such complaint has yet surfaced that dates back to the launching of the FDA's campaign against stevia. However, an "anonymous" trade complaint submitted some time later is indeed on record, one that forced Celestial Seasonings to suspend its use of stevia in its popular line of herbal teas. Was the trade complaint filed by the NutraSweet Company (previously owned by G.D. Searle and now a Monsanto subsidiary), the manufacturer of aspartame? In an article in the August 27, 1996 edition of the *Fresno Bee*, Richard Nelson, vice president of public affairs for NutraSweet, denies that his company had anything to do with the FDA's ban of stevia.

Despite presentations to the FDA of substantial historical and scientific data of stevia safety in petitions submitted in 1992 by the American Herbal Products Association (AHPA)—an association of companies that manufacture and distribute herbal products—and the Thomas J. Lipton Company, seeking GRAS (generally recognized as safe) status for stevia, the FDA refused to consider filing the petitions. (When particular herbs or natural products have been historically in use for a long time, the FDA generally allows them a GRAS status.) In fact, a review of the correspondence between the FDA and representatives from the AHPA, reveals a number of unreasonable requests made by the FDA. These requests caused delays that appeared to be of a stalling nature.

Rob McCaleb, president of the Herb Research Foundation, has, for many years, coordinated the herbal industry's efforts to convince the FDA of stevia's safety. McCaleb says, "The FDA banned stevia from food because of a complaint by a big company (whose name the FDA won't reveal). The FDA has no credible evidence questioning the safety of stevia. This appears to have more to do with protecting profit than public health."

By denying it official GRAS status, the FDA placed stevia in the "food additive" category, which required that it undergo substantial scientific study prior to marketing. The fact that stevia is a sweetener complicates the matter further, since the FDA tends to view any "new" sweetener as an additive with a particularly high potential for mass consumption, necessitating special scrutiny.

In 1994, however, passage of the Dietary Supplement Health and Education Act (DSHEA) created an opportunity for stevia to continue being imported to the United States despite the FDA's opposition. Under this legislation, various vitamins, minerals, herbs, or other botanicals not considered conventional foods or the sole item in a meal or diet may be marketed in the form of capsules, tablets, liquids, powders, or soft gels provided they are labeled "dietary supplements." Such supplements can no longer be classified by the FDA as "food additives," and they do not have to be subjected to intensive safety testing.

In the following fall of 1995, stevia did indeed gain status as a dietary supplement after a seventy-five-day "premarket notification" was submitted to the FDA by a vitamin company. The FDA could have challenged that, too (and still can, for that matter) by claiming that there is inadequate safety information on stevia. Had it done so, however, the FDA would have borne the burden of proof for making such a claim. A lengthy debate would have ensued, leaving them open to the scrutiny of the media and the public. It chose not to pick a fight.

PASS ME THAT LEGAL WHITE POWDER

At long last stevia is legally available in the United States—but only in its limited form as a dietary supplement. Any other use (such as an additive to teas or processed foods) continues to be prohibited if the label claims that the stevia is added for sweetening purposes. Stevia "supplements" cannot be labeled as sweeteners or described as having any kind of sweetening power. Furthermore, no literature mentioning stevia's sweetening ability can be marketed along with the product. Read on.

Déjà Vu in 1998—The FDA and Fahrenheit 451?

As they say, history tends to repeat itself, although in somewhat modified ways. In May of 1998, a compliance officer from the Dallas, Texas, district office of the FDA, sent a fax to Oscar Rodes of Stevita Company, the same stevia marketer whose warehouse had been raided back in 1991. This time, the FDA was disturbed that Rodes was selling the stevia product in conjunction with some literature on stevia, including three books. The law prohibits any literature about a supplement that is not FDA-approved to accompany, or to be in close proximity to that supplement, since the literature could be considered an illegal extension of the product's label.

The letter by the FDA in part reads, "The inspection of your facility on April 27, 1998, conducted jointly by investigators of the FDA and the Texas Department of Health, along with visits to your consignees, documented your firm's continued marketing of your stevia products as conventional foods accompanied by offending [sic] literature, cookbooks, and other publications.

"A current inventory must be taken by an investigator of this office, who will be available to witness destruction of the cookbooks, literature, and other publications for the purpose of verifying compliance."

According to FDA officials, the herb stevia can be "adulterated" merely by being in the presence of information that reveals its sweetening property. Furthermore, the FDA confiscated two shipments of stevia to Rodes from Brazil and asked him to recall the books he had already distributed.

This story was picked up by the media, who strongly criticized the FDA. Pressure mounted. At the end of June of that year, Rodes got a letter from the FDA, who now said that he was allowed to sell two out of the three books along with stevia. One of the cookbooks was not permitted since it mentioned Rodes' product name in the text.

Understandably, it is important to have a law that restricts claims made on labels and accompanying literature regarding the therapeutic use of supplements, since many marketers can make exaggerated or inaccurate claims about the products they sell. However, doesn't it seem silly that it is illegal for a product label to claim that stevia is a sweetener when this fact is so obvious? How can stevia ever fairly compete with aspartame and saccharin when the latter two are allowed to be called sweeteners?

The FDA does have a great burden on its shoulders. After all, it has the responsibility of making sure food products don't have the potential to harm the public. But was its ban on the import of stevia into this country and the subsequent rigid enforcement of existing rules, justified by the published scientific studies, or are there . . . ahem . . . how should we say . . . nonscientific reasons involved?

CHAPTER 3

How Safe Are Sweeteners?

P atent a synthetic sweetener, do some toxicity studies in animals that show it to be safe, send the results to the FDA for their stamp of approval, and you're instantly a billionaire. It's that easy. Actually, even if the artificial sweetener is suspected of causing cancer in animals, and you happen to have a great lobbying team, you can still make your billions. But, if you happen to want to sell a natural product as a sweetener that has been used for centuries and has not been shown to cause toxicity in animals and humans, good luck.

ARTIFICIAL SWEETENERS

There are three major artificial sweeteners sold in this country—saccharin, aspartame, and acesulfame K—and more are on their way. Let's briefly review their safety.

Saccharin

Discovered in 1879, saccharin (the main ingredient in SWEET 'N LOW) is a zero-calorie granulated sugar substitute that is 200 to 400 times sweeter than cane sugar. One .035-ounce packet (1 gram) contains the sweetness of two teaspoons of sugar. Saccharin is often added to soft drinks, gum, toothpaste, and foods such as dietetic canned fruits and salad dressings. SWEET 'N LOW comes in a highly recognized pink packet with the following very serious warning that appears in barely visible letters:

USE OF THIS PRODUCT MAY BE HAZARDOUS TO YOUR HEALTH. THIS PRODUCT CONTAINS SACCHARIN WHICH HAS BEEN DETERMINED TO CAUSE CANCER IN LABORATORY ANIMALS.

Since 1981, after a Canadian study indicated saccharin caused bladder cancer in laboratory animals, it has been listed in the U.S. government's "Report on Carcinogens." On October 31, 1997, the National Institute of Environmental Health—a government advisory panel—recommended that any product containing this sweetener must carry a warning label. An industry group called Calorie Control Council, which had sought a review of the warning, was not happy with this decision. They argued that the studies done on rats were not comparable to those done on humans.

In January 1998, National Cancer Institute researchers announced that saccharin does not cause bladder cancer in monkeys. They tested twenty monkeys for as long as twenty-four years, giving them 25 milligrams of saccharin per kilogram of body weight five days a week. This dose is about five times of that allowed in humans. Sixteen monkeys who received no saccharin served as the control group in the study. Urine testing in the last two years showed no evidence of bladder cancer.

For the time being, the question of saccharin's safety is still debatable. It is not fully known whether long-term saccharin ingestion influences human tumor formation or whether it has any other long-term health consequences.

Aspartame

The main ingredient in NutraSweet and Equal, aspartame was approved by the FDA in 1981 and allowed in diet sodas in 1983. It has no warnings on the packet other than one regarding its use by anyone with phenylketonuria (PKU), a rare inherited condition. Uninformed consumers assume that they can use aspartame without any harmful effects, ingesting it as a sweetener in hundreds of products. NutraSweet's parent company was the pharmaceutical giant G.D. Searle, which was later purchased by Monsanto.

Discovered in 1965 in the course of ulcer drug research, aspartame is comprised of phenylalanine, aspartic acid, and methanol, or wood alcohol, which, when ingested, breaks down into formaldehyde. Aspartame has been the prime suspect in a variety of symptoms chronicled in thousands of consumer complaints to the FDA and the Dallas-based Aspartame Consumer Safety Network. These include gastrointestinal symptoms, headaches, rashes, depression, seizures, memory loss, blurred vision, slurred speech, and other neurological disorders. Of course, just because a person experiences a particular symptom after ingesting a particular substance doesn't automatically make the substance the culprit. It could be just coincidence.

It's very difficult to pinpoint the ingestion of aspartame as the cause of a symptom or disease, since a number of other factors are generally involved. Chemical additives and preservatives in food and beverages, for example, may also be suspect. However, the scientific community is starting to raise some concerns that aspartame may not be as benign as some would have us believe.

At least two scientists, Drs. John Olney and Nuri Farber, from the Department of Psychiatry at the Washington University Medical School in St. Louis, Missouri, believe aspartame to be suspect in a number of physical conditions. In an article published in the November 1996 issue of *Journal of Neuropathology and Experimental Neurology,* they say, "In the past two decades, brain tumor rates have risen in several industrialized countries, including the United States. . . . Compared to other environmental factors putatively linked to brain tumors, the artificial sweetener aspartame is a promising candidate to explain the recent increase in incidence and degree of malignancy of brain tumors. Evidence potentially implicating aspartame includes an early animal study revealing an exceedingly high incidence of brain tumors in aspartame-fed rats compared to no brain tumors in concurrent controls, the recent finding that the aspartame molecule has mutagenic potential, and the close temporal association (aspartame was introduced into U.S. food and beverage markets several years prior to the sharp increase in brain tumor incidence and malignancy). We conclude that there is need for reassessing the carcinogenic potential of aspartame." (Olney, Farber, 1996)

We spoke with Dr. Farber in August of 1997. During our conversation, he reaffirmed their position, "We have not changed our minds and still stand by our conclusions that the carcinogenic potential of aspartame needs to be reassessed."

The FDA issued a statement regarding aspartame in November of 1996. It said, "A recently published medical journal article raises the question whether any increased incidence in the number of persons with brain tumors in the United States is associated with the marketing of aspartame.

"Analysis of the National Cancer Institute's public data base on cancer incidence in the United States does not support an association between the use of aspartame and increased incidence of brain tumors.

"The FDA stands behind its original approval decision, but the Agency remains ready to act if credible scientific evidence is presented to it."

Aspartame, though, does have some advantages. In studies involving laboratory rats, it has been found not to cause tooth cavities (Das, 1997), and its use as a sugar substitute has led to better weight control (Blackburn, 1997). However, similar benefits can also be said of stevia.

In our opinion, the jury on aspartame is still out.

Acesulfame K

Acesulfame K (the K stands for potassium) is better-known by the brand names Sweet One, Swiss Sweet, and Sunette. It is contained in a few commercial products including nondairy creamers, instant coffee and tea, sugar-free puddings, gelatins, chewing gum, and soft drinks. Approved by the FDA in 1988, acesulfame K is a derivative of aceoacetic acid, a synthetic chemical, and is 200 times sweeter than sugar. It is probably not metabolized by the body.

Neither a health warning nor an information label is required for acesulfame K. The benefits or harms of the long-term use of this artificial sweetener in humans is currently not known.

Neotame

With claims that it is 8,000 times sweeter than sugar, neotame is a synthetic sweetener developed by the Monsanto Company, maker of aspartame. In 1998, Monsanto submitted an application to the FDA to market neotame as a tabletop sweetener as well as a sweetening ingredient in foods and beverages. The FDA approval process is expected to last two to three years.

If approved, neotame could replace NutraSweet (Monsanto's brand of aspartame) which has faced intense price competition in major markets because patents that once covered it have expired.

A Final Word on Artificial Sweeteners

As you have seen, the currently available artificial sweeteners, although not proven to be clearly harmful, have not been proven completely safe, either. We believe substituting stevia for saccharin, acesulfame K, and aspartame, even partially, is a reasonable and prudent option for the consumer. Let's take a close look at the stevia safety issue.

STEVIA SAFETY

What about the safety of stevia? To begin with, consider that stevia has been used as a sweetening ingredient in foods and beverages by South American natives for many centuries; it has also been added to a number of food products in Japan since the mid 1970s. To date, there has not been one report of plant toxicity by consumers. Similarly, no incidents of any adverse reactions to stevia have been reported in the United States. Although at this point there have been no indications that stevia is toxic to humans, it is still important that we review the available safety studies done thus far.

Our Daily Stevia Dose

It has been estimated that sugar consumption in Japan is about 80 grams a day, while in the United States and Europe it is between 120 to 140 grams a day (Akashi). If you were to substitute stevia for sugar, what would your daily consumption be?

For the sake of simplicity, let's say you consume about 100 grams of sugar a day. Since the sweetness of stevioside is 300 times that of sugar, simply divide 100 grams by 300. This is one-third of a gram (roughly 330 milligrams). Actually, Chinese researchers have already estimated that the daily human consumption of stevioside is about 2 milligrams per kilogram (mg/kg) of body weight (Xili, 1992). This is a very small amount. It is important to keep this in mind when evaluating the following stevia toxicity studies. Also keep in mind that many people only partially substitute stevia for sugar and other sweeteners. In such cases, the intake of stevia on a daily basis would be even less than 330 milligrams.

There have been a number of studies performed on rodents and other laboratory animals to determine whether stevia has any toxic side effects. In many of these studies, stevia was provided in extremely high dosages, sometimes up to 5 percent of the weight of the animal's food. Let's compare this to humans. Assuming we eat about two kilograms of food a day, and we ingest 200 milligrams of stevia, the proportion of stevia to our daily food intake would be about 0.01 percent—a very small amount, indeed.

Let's examine a few studies done over the past two decades with stevia.

Animal Studies

Whenever researchers want to determine the safety of a substance they begin by testing it on laboratory animals, usually mice or rats. The animals are given a small dose of the substance at the onset of the trial, then they are given progressively higher doses. The increased dosage continues until a lethal dose (LD)—in which 50 percent of the test animals die—is reached. This level is called the LD 50. In the 1970s, several research groups attempted to find the lethal dose of stevia (Kinghorn, 1985). They discovered that, on average, a dose of 8,000 milligrams or more per kilogram of body weight is necessary to achieve the LD 50. This is equivalent to a person weighing 70 kilograms (about 150 pounds) ingesting more than 480,000 milligrams (one pound) of the extract. In most cases, an eight-ounce glass of water can be sweetened with less than four drops of stevia—an extremely small amount. As you might have expected, no human has ever died from stevia overdose.

In a study published in Japan in 1985, researchers determined that giving laboratory rats 550 mg/kg of stevioside every day for two years did not cause any abnormalities. However, the question remained as to whether the ingestion of stevia could cause abnormalities in the offspring.

In 1991, an excellent study was done by researchers at the Chulalongkorn University Primate Research Center in Bangkok, Thailand (Yodyingyuad, 1991). The researchers' objective was to study the consequences of daily ingestion of stevioside—the main active sweetening agent in the stevia plant—in hamsters and its effects on two subsequent generations.

This study involved four groups of twenty hamsters (ten males and ten females) who were one-month-old. Each of the hamsters weighed between 30 and 50 grams. The first group was fed a daily stevioside dosage of 500 mg/kg; the second group received a higher dose at 1,000 mg/kg; and the third group dosage was the highest at 2,500 mg/kg. The fourth group, which served as the control, received no stevioside. To gain a better understanding of just how much stevioside was given to the hamsters, know that a dosage of 2,500 mg/kg given to an average-sized human adult would be approximately 150,000 milligrams (5 ounces). To put this into perspective, know that it is unlikely that any person would ingest more than 500 milligrams of stevia (for sweetening their drinks and certain foods) in any given day. As mentioned earlier, the maximum average stevia intake constitutes approximately 0.01 percent of one's daily food intake.

The study showed no significant difference in the average growth of the first generation of hamsters in the groups receiving stevioside—no matter what dosage they were given. Even the third generation of hamsters, at 120 days of age, showed no significant differences in body weight—no matter which group they were in.

As to the mating performance, all three generations performed the same, no matter which dose of stevioside they received. Their performance was equal to the controls. Microscopic examination of reproductive tissue samples from all of the groups, both male and female, of all of the generations, did not differ from the control group. The production of sperm was normal, even in the males who received the highest dose of stevioside. In the females, the ovaries of all the animals were perfectly normal.

In summary, no growth or fertility abnormalities were found in hamsters of either sex. Mating was efficient and successful. The duration of pregnancies, number of fetuses, as well as number of young delivered each time from females in the experimental groups were not significantly different from those in the control group. The researchers agreed, "The results of this study are astonishing. Stevioside at a dose as high as 2,500 mg/kg did not do any harm to these animals. We conclude that stevioside at a dose as high as 2.5 grams per kilogram (g/kg) of body weight affects neither growth nor reproduction in hamsters. If this is true in other mammalian species including humans, this substance will be of great benefit to industry and medicine, and can be used more widely as a non-caloric sweetener in a variety of foods and drinks, as already seen in Japan and Brazil."

The Latest Safety Study

"Assessment of the carcinogenicity of stevioside in rats," was the title of an article published in the June 1997 issue of *Food and Chemical Toxicology*. We were very excited and anxious when we came across this study. Was this latest information going to show that stevioside was safe or that it was potentially harmful?

The study was performed by Dr. K. Toyoda and colleagues, from the Division of Pathology, National Institute of Health Sciences in Tokyo, Japan. For a period of 104 weeks (two years), three groups of lab rats—fifty male and fifty female—were tested. One group received stevioside in a concentration that constituted 2.5 percent of their daily diets; the second group received a concentration that constituted 5 percent of their diets. The third group, which served as the control, received no stevioside. At the end of the study, all of the surviving rats were euthanized. The rats who received the stevioside weighed less than those in the control group. Considering stevioside has no calories, this makes sense. When the organs and tissues of the rats were examined under a microscope, there was almost no difference between those who were given stevia and those who were not. One interesting difference, however, was that the females who took stevioside had a decreased incidence of breast tumors, while the males displayed a lesser incidence of kidney damage. The researchers state, "It is concluded that stevioside is not carcinogenic in rats under the experimental conditions described."

You may recall at the start of this chapter that we estimated an average person's daily dietary intake of stevioside to be, at most, about 0.01 percent of the total daily intake of food. It is reassuring that rats given significantly higher amounts of this sweetener did not have a greater incidence of tumors than those who did not take the sweetener.

Our interpretation of this research leads us to believe that the small amount of stevioside we may consume daily is extremely safe. Nevertheless, it was banned for import in 1991. Were the reasons justified?

The FDA's Concern

Stevia leaves and extracts were banned from importation in 1991. What was it that prompted the FDA to ban the import of this natural sweetener?

One possible explanation is the result of a 1985 laboratory study that hinted a biochemical breakdown product of stevia to be a possible health concern. This study was conducted at the College of Pharmacy, University of Illinois in Chicago (Pezutto). A strain of a bacterium called *Salmonella typhimurium*—commonly used to determine the toxicity of a substance—was exposed to stevioside. There were no toxic reactions. Many sweet-tasting chemicals related to stevioside were also found to be of no concern. However, steviol, a metabolite, or breakdown product of stevioside, caused some changes in the DNA of this bacteria. It is important to note that this occurred only in the presence of a liquid fraction derived from the livers of rats who had been treated with a chemical called Aroclor 1254, and then exposed to other chemicals. As you can see, this is getting a little complicated and far-fetched. When steviol was given to the bacteria without first being exposed to the above toxins, there were no problems detected.

When humans ingest stevia, their livers are not first damaged by a toxic chemical. It would seem then, at least in our opinion, that the above study has little, if any, relevance to humans and is best ignored in light of the long-term studies with lab animals discussed earlier. Those studies are more practical and relevant. You may recall that when rodents are given stevia in massive doses for at least two generations, no side effects occur.

In case you have any concerns, a study performed in 1993 should comfort you. Researchers from the Department of Biochemistry at Chiang Mai University in Thailand, tested stevioside and steviol for mutagenicity (causing mutation, or changes in the DNA) using a strain of *Salmonella typhimurium* bacteria (Suttajit). The sweeteners were also tested to see their effects on cultured human lymphocytes (types of while blood cells). The bacteria were cultured in a nutrient broth and then placed on a petri dish. Stevioside did not cause any mutations in either of the strains, even when given at concentrations of up to 25 milligrams per dish. When stevioside was given to the bacterial strain at an unusually high dose of 50 milligrams, weak mutagenicity was indicated.

Even more important, no significant chromosomal effects of stevioside and steviol were observed in cultured human blood lymphocytes. The researchers stated, "This study indicates that stevioside and steviol are neither mutagenic nor clastogenic [capable of causing damage to chromosomes] *in vitro* [in a test tube] at the limited doses."

Since the availability of human research on stevia consumption during pregnancy is lacking, it is currently not known if stevia is safe to use during this time or while trying to conceive. Although it would seem extremely unlikely that small amounts of stevia would have any effects on reproduction or the course of pregnancy, until formal human studies are conducted, it would seem prudent for women to use stevia in moderation while they are trying to conceive and during their pregnancies.

IN SUMMARY

One can study the influence of a particular chemical in an isolated petri dish, in a test tube, or on laboratory animals, but not necessarily know what this chemical will do in the human body. After having reviewed all the safety studies published thus far, and considering the safe, centuries-old consumption of stevia in South America, and of its two decades plus use by the Japanese, it is our opinion that stevia is safe for human consumption, particularly in the dosages normally consumed as a partial alternative to artificial sweeteners, as well as sugar and other natural sweeteners.

Having reviewed all of the published studies on stevia that had been available in 1991, we did not encounter any that would justify the great lengths the FDA undertook that year to ban the import of stevia to this country. In our opinion, there seems to be enough evidence to suspect that the FDA, for some reason, was biased against stevia.

CHAPTER 4

The Many Faces of Stevia—Leaves, Powder, and Liquid

Stevia, which is now permitted on the market as a dietary supplement as long as it is not labeled a sweetener and poised to become an extremely popular product, is available in a variety of different forms. It comes in leaves—both fresh and dried—powder, and liquid. The product you choose is likely to depend on what you are using it for.

A number of manufacturers produce stevia in its many forms. This is why each stevia product may taste slightly different. For instance, you may find the white extract from one manufacturer to have a slight licorice aftertaste, while a different brand may have no aftertaste at all. Don't give up on stevia if you expect it to have the exact sweetness of sugar. It doesn't. However, it's close, and when you consider the wonderful benefits it provides, you may accept its slight imperfections. For some people, stevia, just like wine, is an acquired taste.

Let's take a closer look at the different forms in which stevia is available. Most products are found in health food stores, although a growing number of grocery stores and retail outlets are also beginning to stock stevia products on their shelves.

FRESH LEAVES

Stevia's most natural, unrefined state is in its fresh leaf form. As discussed earlier, for many centuries, the Guarani Indians of South America have used fresh stevia leaves to sweeten their drinks. They discovered chewing on a leaf picked from a stevia plant will impart a long-lasting, extremely sweet taste sensation that is reminiscent of licorice. In Bertoni's first official description of the stevia plant, he noted that, "A fragment of the leaf suffices to keep the mouth sweet for an hour."

As it is difficult to grow stevia from seeds, a number of companies sell cuttings (check your local health food store for such companies, or do a search on the internet). You can purchase some cuttings and plant them yourself in your own home or yard. Stevia thrives outdoors in hot, sunny weather, and does equally well in an indoor window garden. Just one word of caution: If you own a cat, you may not have too many stevia leaves left. They love to chew on them.

DRIED LEAVES

You can find whole dried stevia leaves in health food stores. To release the flavor and sweetness of the leaves, crushing is necessary. A dried leaf is considerably sweeter than a fresh one, and it is the form of stevia commonly used to sweeten herbal tea. When added to herbal tea blends, amounts can be adjusted to provide more or less of a sweet taste. Finely powdered or pulverized stevia leaves can also be purchased in bulk form. Several tea manufacturers add the pulverized leaves and other herbs to their tea bags. Of course, because of the FDA ruling, they are not permitted to mention that the stevia is for sweetening purposes. Instead, stevia is labeled as a dietary supplement.

Stevia leaves, which are greenish in color, can be used as flavor enhancers or sweeteners in a wide variety of foods and beverages such as vegetable dishes, coffee and tea, applesauce, and hot cereals. Generally two to four dried leaves are sufficient for sweetening a cup of tea or coffee. However, in this form, expect stevia to have a more noticeable licorice-type aftertaste.

As a rule, about 5 to 10 percent of each leaf contains stevioside and rebaudioside, the actual sweet glycosides of stevia. Although stevia leaves contain various vitamins, minerals, and phytochemicals, the amounts consumed are generally so minimal that their nutritional value is probably negligible.

GREEN STEVIA POWDER

When the dried stevia leaves are ground, they become a fine green powder that is generally about ten to twenty times as sweet as sugar. This powder can be added directly to tea or other dishes. You can also convert this powder into syrup by dissolving 1 teaspoon of the powder into 2 cups of filtered or distilled water. Bring the mixture to a gentle boil, then lower the heat and simmer until it has been reduced to a slightly thick syrup. Once the liquid has cooled, place it in a small bottle, and store it in the refrigerator for increased shelf life.

Generally speaking, green stevia powder is not very popular due to its somewhat strong aftertaste. However, it is available in health food stores. The majority of stevia recipes, including the ones in this book, call for white stevia extract or clear liquid stevia; both have very little or no aftertaste. Always make sure to use the right form.

WHITE STEVIA EXTRACT

White stevia extract, which is actually a powder, is the form most commonly used in Japan. It generally contains 85 to 95 percent of the sweet glycosides. Nearly 300 times sweeter than sugar, white stevia extract has sweetening power that is equivalent to two to four cups of sugar.

Walk into any Japanese restaurant, and there is a good chance that you will find small packets of stevia served along with tea. As only a very tiny amount of the extract is needed, these packets are commonly bulked up with a filler, such as maltodextrin. One company in the United States has also started marketing stevia in small packets to which maltodextrin similarly has been added. Could stevia some day become so popular in the U.S. that restaurants begin offering packets of this sweetener alongside the typical pink packets of SWEET 'N LOW and blue packets of Equal?

There are hundreds of patents worldwide for the extraction of white stevia extract—Japan itself has over 150. Although white ste-via extract has the least noticeable aftertaste of all of the different forms, Canadian researchers are working on an extraction process that *completely* eliminates any aftertaste. This type of extraction would influence the concentration of the various sweet glycosides, such as stevioside and rebaudioside. At this point, Stevia powders are not the same.

Since extracted white stevia powder is so intensely sweet, we recommend that it be mixed with water and used by the drop. See the following information on liquid concentrates for instructions on how to make your own.

LIQUID CONCENTRATES

There are two distinctly different kinds of liquid stevia concen-trate. One is dark and syrupy, the other is clear.

To make the dark concentrate, bring two cups of purified water to a boil. Reduce the heat to medium and add one-half ounce of crushed dried stevia leaves. Cover the pot and boil for three min-utes. Remove the pot from the heat and allow the liquid to steep until cool. Strain the greenish-black liquid through a cheesecloth and refrigerate it in a covered glass jar or container. This, its crud-est form, is the most medicinal way to take stevia for positive effects on the pancreas. It has antifungal and antibacterial proper-ties as well, and can be used topically on skin to treat burns, wounds, and athlete's foot.

To make the clear concentrate—the type most popularly used to sweeten foods and beverages—simply dissolve 1 teaspoon of white stevia powder in 3 tablespoons of filtered or sterile water. Store the liquid, also called a *working solution*, in a dropper-type bottle in the refrigerator. Commercial varieties of this liquid are made by mixing the white powder in distilled water or grain alco-hol. Some of these commercial liquid preparations contain other ingredients such as chrysanthemum flowers.

All types of liquid extract concentrates are commonly available in health food stores. They come in various sized dropper-style bottles, ranging in size from under an ounce to four ounces. Generally, a few drops of this concentrate are enough to sweeten a glass of iced tea or lemonade, a cup of coffee, or just about any other beverage.

A FAMILIAR FACE

A common sight on health food store shelves, stevia, in its many forms, is soon likely to be a familiar face in grocery stores and pharmacies, as well.

CHAPTER 5

Staying Healthy the Stevia Way

Most people have at least an occasional craving for something sweet, and they often satisfy this desire with sugar-laden, fat-filled, foods. One of the biggest problems with sugar is that it can markedly elevate blood sugar levels, throwing off the body's delicate chemical balance. Addictive in nature, sugar also leaches important minerals from the body, causing weakness to the immune system. And any excess sugar is converted by the body into fat. Artificial sugar alternatives such as saccharin and aspartame are certainly not the complete answer, considering their health risks are not fully known (see Chapter 3). So how can that sweet tooth be satisfied without compromising good health? The answer may lie in stevia, nature's calorie-free sweetener.

Although anyone can benefit from using stevia instead of sugar or chemical sugar substitutes, there are certain people who are more likely to benefit from its remarkable sweetening potential. Some of these people include those with diabetes, those interested in decreasing caloric intake, and children.

A GODSEND TO THOSE WITH DIABETES

If you have diabetes, chances are you consume a large amount of artificial sweeteners. Until now, these sweeteners have been the only sugar alternative for those with diabetes. The problem, however, is that there has always been a concern that overconsumption of these synthetic sweeteners may cause some harm to the body. Could partial or complete stevia substitution for artificial sweeteners be a good idea? We believe so. Stevia leaves have been used as herbal teas by diabetic patients in Asian countries for many years. No side effects have been observed in these patients after continued consumption (Suttajit, 1993). Furthermore, studies have shown that stevia extract can actually improve blood sugar levels (Alvarez, 1981, Curi, 1986).

In 1986, Brazilian researchers from the Universities of Maringa and Sao Paolo evaluated the role of stevia in blood sugar (Curi, 1986). Sixteen healthy volunteers were given extracts from 5 grams of stevia leaves every six hours for three days. The extracts were prepared by immersing the leaves in boiling water for twenty minutes. A glucose tolerance test (GTT) was performed before and after the administration of the extract. During this test, the volunteers were given a glass of water with glucose. Blood sugar levels were then evaluated over the next few hours. The results were compared to those of another group of volunteers that did not receive the stevia extracts. Those with a predisposition to diabetes showed marked rise in blood sugar levels. The group given stevia was found to have significantly lower blood sugar levels as indicated by the glucose tolerance tests.

The results of this study were a positive indication that, potentially, stevia can be beneficial to diabetics. And even if stevia by itself does not lower blood sugar levels, the simple fact that a person with diabetes would consume less sugar is of significant importance in maintaining better blood sugar control.

We suggest that switch to stevia. You can begin by using it instead of sugar or an artificial sweetener to flavor your coffee or tea. After a few days or weeks, as your comfort level with stevia increases, gradually use more of the herbal extract in those dishes or beverages in which you would normally use a different sweetener. With time, more research will become available on the safety of stevia and artificial sweeteners. Based on the results of these studies, you can better determine which sweeteners to continue using in greater amounts.

Although some argue that artificial sweeteners are safe in small amounts, problems may arise if they are used in excess. Even partially substituting stevia for artificial sweeteners can help reduce any potential risk.

STEVIA AND WEIGHT LOSS

It would seem quite obvious that even partially substituting a no-calorie sweetener for sugar would help reduce caloric intake and thus contribute to weight loss. (One ounce—approximately 2 teaspoons—of sugar contains 50 calories. The average daily sugar intake for persons in the United States is 13 ounces, or 650 calories.) Such is the case with artificial sweeteners such as aspartame.

Researchers at the Center for the Study of Nutrition Medicine, Beth Israel Deaconess Medical Center at Harvard Medical School in Boston, Massachusetts, studied the influence of aspartame on obesity (Blackburn, 1997). In one study, 163 women were randomly divided into two groups. Each group was assigned to either consume or abstain from aspartame-sweetened foods and beverages for sixteen weeks. Both groups were also actively involved in a weight-control program using a variety of modalities. At the end of the study, both the group on aspartame and the group without the synthetic sweetener lost an average of 10 kilograms (22 pounds). During the maintenance phase that lasted for the next two years, the women assigned to the aspartame group gained back an average of 4.5 kilograms (10 pounds) while those who were not on aspartame gained back 9.4 kilograms (20 pounds)—practically all of the weight they had previously lost. The researchers concluded, "These data suggest that participation in a multidisciplinary weight-control program that includes aspartame may facilitate the long-term maintenance of reduced body weight."

Unfortunately, no formal studies have been done to evaluate stevia substitution in relation to weight loss. However, as stevia has virtually no calories, we would suspect the results to be similar to those in the aspartame study.

Are you the type of person who uses a lot of sugar? Do you use it to sweeten beverages? Do you sprinkle it on cereal? Do you consume it in baked goods and other sweet treats? If so, there's a good possibility that even partially substituting these refined sugar calories with calorie-free stevia can make a difference in your weight.

STEVIA AND TOOTH DECAY

Even a five-year-old child knows that sugar can cause tooth decay. There are certain bacteria in your mouth, particularly *Streptococci mutans*, that ferment various sugars and produce acids. These acids, in turn, eat through the enamel of the tooth, causing a decayed spot or cavity. For a long time, scientists have searched to find alternative sweeteners that are not fermentable by bacteria and, hence, do not cause cavities. Artificial sweeteners have been helpful in this regard.

Does stevia lead to tooth cavities? According to one study done on laboratory rats, the answer is no. In this study, stevioside and rebaudioside A—the two primary sweet constituents of the stevia plant—were tested on a group of sixty rat pups (Das, 1992). The rats were divided into four groups. Group 1 was fed 30 percent of its diet in sucrose (table sugar). Group 2 was given 0.5 percent of its diet in stevioside. Group 3 received 0.5 percent of its diet in rebaudioside A. Group 4, the control group, was given no sugar or sweetener of any kind. There was no difference in the food or water intake among the groups.

After five weeks, the rats were evaluated. There was a significant difference in the condition of their teeth. The sugar-fed rats in Group 1 had significantly more cavities than the rats in the other groups. The rats in Groups 2, 3, and 4 had about the same number of cavities. The researchers stated, "It was concluded that neither stevioside nor rebaudioside A is cariogenic [cavity causing] under the conditions of this study." It appears that the chemicals within the stevia plant that impart its sweetness are not fermentable, and thus do not cause tooth cavities.

CHILDREN AND STEVIA

Candies, sodas, ice cream, pies, cakes . . . It's disturbing how many sugar-sweetened products are consumed by children on a daily basis. As you have seen, sugar is implicated in tooth decay and obesity. Artificial sweeteners, which have other potential long-term health consequences, are not the complete answer.

Certainly, limiting your child's intake of sugary products is strongly suggested. Another option is substituting stevia for sugar wherever possible. For instance, instead of sweetening that glass of ice cold lemonade with sugar or aspartame, use a few drops of stevia instead. Or try substituting stevia for the sugar in your oatmeal cookies. We believe that even partially substituting sugar with stevia can help satisfy your child's sweet tooth while decreasing his or her risks from excessive sugar intake.

Be sure to take advantage of the many recipes provided in Part Two of this book. You will find plenty of tasty treats that will satisfy your child's sweet tooth (and yours, too) without the possible harms of sugar or chemical sugar substitutes.

Eventually, and hopefully soon, stevia will be used in this country as an added ingredient in a variety of commercial products such as soda, candy, chewing gum, prepared foods, and baked goods. It has been a successful addition to such products in Japan for the last two decades.

STEVIA AND HIGH BLOOD PRESSURE

In 1991, Dr. M.S. Melis, from the Department of Biology at the University of Sao Paulo in Brazil, did a study to determine the effects of stevioside on blood pressure. After giving a one-time high-dose injection of stevioside to a group of laboratory rats, he found that they experienced a reduction in blood pressure as well as an increased elimination of sodium (Melis, 1991). A slight diuretic effect also occurred. The effect was even stronger when stevia was combined with verapamil, a medicine commonly prescribed for lowering blood pressure.

In a similar study in 1995, Dr. Melis administered oral doses of stevia to lab rats for up to sixty days. After twenty days, there were no changes in the stevia-treated rats compared to those who did not receive the extract. However, after both forty and sixty days of administering the stevia, the rats showed reduction in blood pressure, a diuretic effect, and an increase in sodium loss. The amount of blood going to the kidneys was also increased. (Melis, 1991).

One small study in Brazil involved eighteen average, healthy human volunteers between the ages of twenty and forty years. After the test subjects were given tea prepared with stevia leaves for thirty days, a 10-percent lowering of blood pressure occurred (Boeck, 1981). Although this study gives an indication of stevioside's effects on lowering blood pressure, certainly more human studies are needed before we can know the full vascular effects of stevia consumption.

STEVIA AND PREGNANT OR BREASTFEEDING WOMEN

No human studies involving stevia and pregnant or breastfeeding women have been conducted at this point in time. As a result, we do not know with certainty whether its use during this period is safe. Although we suspect that small amounts of stevia will not cause any problems in these women, we cannot say for sure.

STEVIA'S ANTI-AGING POTENTIAL

We know from numerous animal studies that reducing caloric intake can be a factor in extending lifespan. We know that excess amounts of calorie-laden sugar can contribute to high blood sugar, obesity, and a number of other unhealthy side effects, including aging.

Glucose (sugar) has been implicated in the aging process by its ability to react with some proteins, like collagen, to produce glycation. That is, the glucose molecule attaches to some amino acids of a protein and makes the protein less functional, leading to disturbances within a cell. The initial phase of this attachment is called glycation.

As we age, the amount of glycation of the proteins in our bodies tends to increase. We should also note that blood sugar generally increases as we age. It is known that glycation of human tendon and aortic collagen increases with age in proportion to the increase in blood glucose that occurs with aging (Schleicher, 1996 and 1997).

This age-related increase in glycation, though, can be partially prevented by caloric restriction. In other words, avoiding high sugar and high calorie consumption could, theoretically, over the years and decades, help our proteins stay healthier.

CONCLUSION

Although, at this time, the therapeutic potential of stevia has not been fully determined, a number of positive effects have been indicated. Partial substitution of stevia for sugar can have a positive effect on blood sugar. Stevia is helpful for those with diabetes, those interested in reducing their caloric intake, and those interested in reducing sugar-related tooth decay. It also promotes general good health and longevity.

CHAPTER 6

Cooking
With Stevia

Our health would be greatly enhanced if we could reduce the amount of sugar we consume, especially refined sugar. At four calories per gram, basically void of any nutrients, with a fantastic ability to raise blood sugar and stimulate a wicked insulin response, you're better off not even walking near the aisle where sugar is shelved at your local grocery store. If you already have an unopened bag at home, consider using it for something useful—say, a doorstop. Sure, we're being a bit harsh on sugar. Other than its sweet taste, it does have some assets, which we'll discuss later, that have contributed to its overwhelming popularity with chefs and bakers.

Fortunately, with the availability of stevia, we can greatly reduce or completely avoid our consumption of white refined sugar. By blending stevia with high-quality, healthier sweet products (such as mineral-rich natural sugars like molasses, barley malt, fruit juices, rice syrup, and honey), we can still have delicious low- or no-refined-sugar meals and treats.

We're confident that you will find stevia's sweetness just as appealing as sugar in most recipes. With only a few exceptions, the recipes in this book use stevia as their exclusive sweetening agent. In the few recipes that are only partially sweetened with stevia, the original sugar amount has been greatly reduced. For instance, the

French Chocolate Ice Cream recipe found on page 136 originally called for one cup of sugar. We discovered that by adding a tiny amount of stevia, we were able to reduce the sugar volume to one-quarter cup and still have a delicious dessert. As you try these recipes, you may choose to follow them exactly, or you may wish to use stevia in combination with other sweeteners if you prefer.

A growing number of chefs throughout the country are creating a wonderful variety of smoothies and other beverages, baked goods, sorbets, ice creams, puddings, and even stevia-sweetened cheesecakes for their clientele. The R. Thomas Deluxe Grille, in Atlanta, Georgia, for instance, makes an organic butternut squash pie topped with whipped cream—both sweetened with stevia—that is extremely popular with its health-conscious patrons. You can take pride in joining those who are working to offer Americans healthier, higher quality sweets without sacrificing taste.

When you start cooking and baking with stevia, you will find that it has a number of advantageous characteristics, as well as some minor drawbacks. Let's discuss some of these characteristics now.

ADVANTAGES

In addition to adding sweetness to foods and beverages, in many cases, stevia serves as a flavor enhancer. When added to lemon juice, for example, stevia clearly heightens the flavor of the lemon. When it is used in a peach cobbler, the peach flavor really stands out. And the addition of stevia to homemade ice cream gives the ice cream an even creamier texture. Another beauty of stevia is that it is capable of remaining stable when combined with acidic foods. It can successfully sweeten dishes that include tomatoes and most fruits.

One more wonderful characteristic of stevia is that high temperatures do not destroy its sweetening properties. It neither ferments, nor does it discolor. This means you can use stevia in hot dishes as well as in baked goods. The artificial sweetener aspartame cannot make such a claim.

STEVIA IS NOT PERFECT

As advantageous as stevia is, it does have a few minor drawbacks. For instance, foods baked with stevia do not rise as well as those baked with sugar. In addition to contributing sweetness, sugar has a crystalline structure that provides texture to baked goods. It also aids in the creaming and whipping process during mixing. Sugar helps create softening or spreading action to batter, and it caramelizes, which enhances browning. Sugar also feeds the fermentation of yeast and retains moisture. Stevia is not suitable for these purposes.

Some users of stevia are sensitive to the slight aftertaste. (Artificial sweeteners such as aspartame and saccharin also have a noticeable aftertaste.) We've found, however, that baking or cooking usually eliminates this taste. As you experiment with different brands of stevia, you may find slight differences in both sweetness and aftertaste. Try at least two or three different products to identify the one that you find most suitable.

The green stevia powder may slightly change the color of your food. You can avoid this by using the white powdered extract instead. The recipes in this book call for the white stevia powder or the liquid concentrate made from that powder.

PRACTICAL TIPS AND SUGGESTIONS

Those who are novices at using stevia often make the same mistake—they use too much of it. Since stevia is up to 300 times sweeter than sugar, excessive amounts can lead to over-sweetness and an aftertaste. For instance, when Dr. Sahelian's mom made the Currant Oatmeal Cookies, found on page 128, she made two separate batches. In one batch, she used the exact amount of stevia called for in the recipe—$^3/_4$ teaspoon. To the second batch, she added 1 full teaspoon. The first batch was delicious, while the second batch had a mild, but noticeable, aftertaste.

At first, stevia's flavor may take a little getting used to. It might be a good idea to mix it with even a tiny amount of another sweetener like honey, which usually eliminates any aftertaste. When combined with another sweetener, stevia usually takes a second position in flavor, but definitely increases the product's sweetness.

When creating new recipes in your own kitchen, it is important to know that stevia's unique sweetness is often more noticeable when used with neutral or mild-flavored foods. So be careful. The smallest amount can overpower the food's original flavor. Stevia's taste is not as apparent in strong or bitter-tasting foods like coffee or unsweetened cocoa, but it blends especially well with citrus flavors such as lemon and cranberry. Stevia is delicious with dairy foods (yogurt, cream, ice cream, kefir), as well as with chocolate and carob. Most fruits also go very well with stevia. If you are one of the millions of Americans who have a love affair with chocolate, you'll be delighted to know that stevia and chocolate (or carob), especially with a little fresh organic cream, are perfect partners.

Unless otherwise specified, always add stevia, in both powder and liquid forms, to the liquid ingredients of a recipe. And when adapting a favorite recipe by substituting sugar with stevia, keep in mind that you may need to increase slightly the amount of liquid (egg, water, milk) that is called for. Just be careful with those eggs, though. While eggs do help provide the "rise" or leavening to baked goods, too many eggs can "toughen" your finished product.

In creating the recipes for this book, we found our greatest challenge was with cakes. Flour, having a slightly bitter nature, is not as delicious with stevia as it is when combined with sugar. During our experimenting, we found that adding ingredients like grated lemon peel and nuts helped improve the cake's flavor. Achieving a light, fluffy texture was a little more difficult. We found single-layer cakes to be the best. They could be enjoyed as is, or stacked on top of one another with various kinds of icings in between. In our muffin recipes, generally we suggest mini muffins, which seem to rise better than the standard-sized variety.

BAKING WITH STEVIA

As mentioned above, baked goods sweetened solely with stevia do not brown as well as those made with sugar. (The exceptions are those products made with chocolate or carob, which lend a rich brown color.) It is for this reason we suggest decorating your cakes and muffins with some fresh fruit, a creamy frosting, or a dollop of whipped cream. This will give the items a more eye-appealing presentation.

Because of this lack of browning ability, you must rely on your sense of touch and smell when checking to see if your muffins and cakes are done. When your kitchen is filled with that wonderful "bakery" smell, open your oven door and gently poke the cake to see if it is "springy" to the touch. Or insert a toothpick into its center. If the toothpick comes out clean, you'll know the cake is done.

We do not recommend stevia as the sole sweetener in yeasted breads or cakes. Sugar is necessary to activate yeast's rising power.

STEVIA CONVERSION RATE

Let's say you've decided to substitute stevia for the sugar in some of your favorite recipes. How do you determine the amount to use? Unfortunately, we can't give you an exact answer for several reasons. Very sour foods like cranberries and lemons need more sweetener than a pie baked with apples or pears, which are naturally sweet. Then there's personal preference. Some people like their foods sweeter than others. There's also a cultural difference. As a rule, Americans like their foods sweet.

To complicate matters even further, there are a number of different companies that make stevia. The quality, flavor, and sweetness varies from product to product. Your best option is to try a few different brands and choose the one you like best. Some companies combine pure stevia powder with maltodextrin or another filler. While such products are still sweet, they don't compare in strength to the pure powder. The stevia powder called for in this book's recipes is the pure form.

Although different stevia products offer different levels of sweetness, we have provided approximate stevia equivalencies. When substituting stevia for sugar, use the following chart to determine proper amounts. Remember, these equivalents are *approximate.*

If you are new to cooking with stevia, always start with either the exact amount called for in the recipe, or a little less. Then taste the batter, sauce, salad dressing, smoothie, or whatever you are

Sugar Amount	Equivalent Stevia Powdered Extract	Equivalent Stevia Liquid Concentrate
1 cup	1 teaspoon	1 teaspoon
1 tablespoon	$\frac{1}{4}$ teaspoon	6 to 9 drops
1 teaspoon	A pinch to $\frac{1}{16}$ teaspoon	2 to 4 drops

preparing to see if it's sweet enough before adding more. As a general rule, add both liquid and powdered forms of stevia to the liquid portion of the recipe.

When you need only the smallest amount of sweetener to flavor a cup of tea or coffee, for example, you may find the stevia powder a little difficult to adjust. Even the tiny amount you may gather onto the point of a dinner knife might make that cup of tea or coffee too sweet. For this reason, we recommend turning the powder into a "working solution." Dissolve one teaspoon of white powder in three tablespoons of filtered water. Pour the solution into a dropper-style bottle and refrigerate. You can also buy ready-made stevia liquid concentrate from your local health food store.

TIME TO GET STARTED

Almost all of us have a sweet tooth. Wouldn't it be great if we could satisfy that sweet tooth at a fraction of the caloric intake?

As you will see from the many recipes in this book, using stevia as the sole sweetener in pies, puddings, candies, and fruit treats always meets with successful results. When it comes to sweetening cakes, muffins, and other baked goods, however, some people may prefer to use sugar for its contribution to the product's texture and rise. Know that stevia alone can be used in such products with comparable results, and even partially substituting stevia for sugar in baked goods is yet another option.

Substituting calorie-free stevia for sugar, even partially, can be a significant health improvement. Ingesting even 100 less calories a day over the period of a year can result in the loss of quite a few pounds of excess weight. Nearly all of the recipes in the following chapters—including the baked goods—are successfully sweetened with stevia only.

In addition to the recipes in this book, try substituting stevia for the sugar in your own favorite recipes. And if you have diabetes and typically use artificial sweeteners, simply use stevia instead. It is a healthy, natural alternative.

PART TWO

SO LONG, SUGAR

FAVORITE STEVIA RECIPES

STEVIA

SUNRISE

BREAKFASTS

Autumn Apple Crepes

Yield: Four 8-inch crepes

CREPES
$\frac{1}{2}$ cup all-purpose flour
$\frac{1}{4}$ cup water
$\frac{1}{4}$ cup heavy cream
1 large egg
1 egg yolk
6 tablespoons melted butter, or coconut oil
1 tablespoon vanilla flavoring
Pinch sea salt

FILLING
2 tablespoons unsalted butter
$\frac{1}{4}$ cup finely chopped Vidalia or other sweet onion
2 Granny Smith or Golden apples, peeled, cored, and thinly sliced
$\frac{1}{2}$ cup lemon juice
1 tablespoon grated lemon rind
$\frac{1}{8}$ teaspoon white stevia powder, or 8 to 10 drops liquid concentrate

1. To make the crepe batter, place the flour in a medium-sized bowl and slowly whisk in the water and cream until smooth and well blended. Pour the mixture through a fine sieve to remove any lumps, then whisk in the eggs, butter, vanilla, and salt. Cover and let rest at least 1 hour in the refrigerator.

2. Heat an 8-inch, heavy-duty nonstick crepe pan or skillet over medium heat for 30 to 40 seconds, or until a few drops of water bounce and sizzle on the surface.

3. Brush the pan lightly with melted butter, then spoon $\frac{1}{4}$ cup of batter into the center. Tilt the pan in all directions so the batter completely covers the bottom in a thin layer. Pour out any excess.

4. Cook about 30 seconds, or until the bottom of the crepe is lightly browned and can be lifted easily from the pan. Using a fork or your fingers, carefully turn the crepe over.

5. Cook another 15 to 20 seconds, then transfer the crepe to a clean plate to cool. Continue making crepes with the remaining batter.

6. To make filling, melt the butter in a medium-sized skillet over medium heat. Add the onion and apples, and sauté for about 5 minutes or until the apples are soft and the onion is beginning to caramelize. Combine the lemon juice, lemon rind, and stevia in a small bowl, then add it to the apple/onion mixture. Mix well.

7. Spoon 3 tablespoons of filling in the middle of each crepe, then roll up. Serve hot, either as is, or topped with Sweet Whipped Cream (page 103).

HOT BREAKFAST PORRIDGE

Yield: Two 1½-cup servings

2 cups water
1 cup quick-cooking oat flakes or quinoa flakes
¼ teaspoon sea salt
1 teaspoon cinnamon
12 drops stevia liquid concentrate
1 tablespoon butter, or coconut oil
2 teaspoons vanilla flavoring
1 teaspoon flaxseed oil (optional)

1. Place the water in a 1-quart pot and bring to a boil over medium-high heat. Add the oat flakes, salt, cinnamon, stevia, and butter, and reduce the heat to very low. Simmer for 10 minutes.

2. Remove the pot from the heat and allow the oatmeal to cool slightly before adding the vanilla and flaxseed oil, if using. Serve hot.

OLD FASHIONED PANCAKES

*Be sure to top these light, fluffy pancakes with some
stevia-sweetened Maple Syrup (page 103).*

Yield: 14 to 16 pancakes (5 inch)   CUT IN HALF

3/4 cup 1½ cups sifted all-purpose flour

1 teaspoon sea salt

1 tsp 1¾ teaspoons double-acting baking powder

1 3 eggs

1½ 3 tablespoons ~~melted butter~~ oil (coconut oil)

1 cup 2 cups milk

½ to ¼ teaspoon stevia liquid concentrate, or to taste

in dry ingredients

1. In a large mixing bowl, sift together the flour, salt, and baking powder.

2. In a medium-sized mixing bowl, beat the eggs. Add the butter, milk, and stevia, and continue to beat until well-combined.

3. Add the liquid mixture to the dry ingredients and mix until just combined. Do not overmix.

4. Lightly butter a nonstick griddle and place over medium-high heat. Heat the griddle until a few drops of water bounce and sizzle on the surface.

5. Ladle ¼-cup portions of batter onto the griddle. To assure well-rounded pancakes, don't drop the batter from high above, rather let it pour onto the griddle from the side of the ladle.

6. Cook about 1 to 2 minutes, or until bubbles appear on the surface and the bottoms are golden brown. Flip the pancakes over and brown the other side. Serve hot.

Variations

- Nuts, fruits, seeds, and even leftover grains can be added to this basic recipe.

- For wheat-free pancakes, use 1½ cups rice flour, or a combination of ¾ cup amaranth flour and ¾ cup tapioca flour.

HIGH-FIBER WHEAT-FREE PANCAKES

Yield: 12 pancakes (5 inch)

1 cup wheat-free, all-purpose baking mix*
2 heaping tablespoons ground flaxseed
1 tablespoon cinnamon
2 eggs
2 tablespoons melted butter, or coconut oil
$1^1/_2$ cups water, or 1 cup water plus $^1/_2$ cup heavy cream
$^1/_4$ teaspoon stevia liquid concentrate, or to taste
1 tablespoon vanilla flavoring

* Arrowhead Mills brand is recommended.

1. In a large mixing bowl, sift together the baking mix, flaxseed, and cinnamon.

2. In a medium-sized mixing bowl, beat the eggs. Add the butter, water, stevia, and vanilla, and mix until well combined.

3. Add the liquid mixture to the dry ingredients and mix until just combined. Do not overmix.

4. Lightly butter a nonstick griddle and place over medium-high heat. Heat the griddle until a few drops of water bounce and sizzle on the surface.

5. Ladle $^1/_4$-cup portions of batter onto the griddle. To assure well-rounded pancakes, don't drop the batter from high above, rather let it pour onto the griddle from the side of the ladle.

6. Cook about 1 to 2 minutes, or until bubbles appear on the surface and the bottoms are golden brown. Flip the pancakes over and brown the other side. Serve hot.

BUTTERMILK WAFFLES

Stevia-sweetened Maple Syrup (page 103) is the perfect topping for these melt-in-your-mouth waffles.

Yield: 6 standard waffles

2 cups all-purpose flour
1½ teaspoons double-acting baking powder
¼ teaspoon baking soda
½ teaspoon sea salt
2 egg yolks
6 to 9 drops stevia liquid concentrate
1⅔ cups buttermilk, or kefir
6 tablespoons melted butter
2 egg whites

1. Preheat a standard-sized waffle iron.

2. In a large mixing bowl, sift together the flour, baking powder, baking soda, and salt.

3. In a medium-sized bowl, beat the egg yolks and stevia together well. Add the buttermilk and butter, and continue to beat until well combined.

4. Add the liquid mixture to the dry ingredients and mix together with a few swift strokes. Do not overmix.

5. Using an electric hand mixer, beat the egg whites until stiff, then fold them into the batter.

6. When the iron is ready, add enough batter to cover about two-thirds of the grill's surface and close the lid. Cook about 4 minutes, or until steam stops escaping from the sides of the iron. Lift up the cover and remove the waffle.* Repeat with the remaining batter.

* If you lift the top of the iron and the waffle shows resistance, cook the waffle a little longer, then try again.

BANANA-BLUEBERRY MINI MUFFINS

Yield: 24 mini muffins

2 cups all-purpose flour
1 tablespoon baking soda
2 ripe, medium-sized bananas
¼ teaspoon white stevia powder
1 cup buttermilk, or kefir
8 tablespoons unsalted (sweet) butter, melted
2 large egg whites
1 cup blueberries
1 cup chopped walnuts

1. Preheat the oven to 400°F.

2. In a large bowl, sift together the flour and baking soda, and set aside.

3. In a medium-sized bowl, mash the bananas with a fork until they reach a lumpy consistency. Add the stevia to the buttermilk, and combine with the bananas. Gently stir in the melted butter.

5. Using an electric hand-held mixer, beat the egg whites until stiff, then fold them into the banana mixture.

6. Add the banana mixture to the dry ingredients and stir until just mixed. Do not overstir. Gently fold in the blueberries and walnuts.

7. Spoon the batter into a lightly oiled or papered mini muffin tin. Fill each cup with a heaping tablespoon of batter, and bake for about 12 minutes. When a toothpick inserted into the center of a muffin comes out clean, the muffins are done.

CHOCOLATE MINI MUFFINS

Yield: 24 mini muffins

1 cup all-purpose flour
½ cup rice flour
½ cup cocoa powder
1 teaspoon baking powder
¼ teaspoon sea salt
1 tablespoon Dacopa or other instant grain coffee substitute
2 large eggs
½ cup chocolate milk
¼ cup buttermilk, or kefir
1 teaspoon vanilla flavoring
1 tablespoon stevia liquid concentrate
3 tablespoons unrefined, organic safflower or coconut oil*
¼ cup cold butter, thinly sliced
2 cups chopped walnuts or pecans

* You can use ½ cup cold butter, thinly sliced, instead.

1. Preheat the oven to 350°F.

2. In a medium mixing bowl, sift together the all-purpose flour, rice flour, cocoa powder, baking powder, salt, and instant coffee.

3. In a small mixing bowl, combine the eggs, chocolate milk, buttermilk, vanilla, and stevia.

4. Using a fork, work the oil and butter into the dry ingredients.

5. Add the wet ingredients to the dry ingredients, and stir until just mixed. Do not overstir. Fold in the nuts.

6. Spoon the batter into a lightly oiled or papered mini muffin tin. Fill each cup with a heaping tablespoon of batter, and bake for about 12 minutes. When a toothpick inserted into the center of a muffin comes out clean, the muffins are done.

SWEET CORN MINI MUFFINS

Yield: 24 mini muffins

---

1 cup brown rice baking mix*
1 egg, slightly beaten
¾ cup milk
2 tablespoons coconut oil
1 tablespoon liquid stevia concentrate
1 to 2 cups fresh corn kernels

* Fern's brand is recommended; however, you can substitute this ingredient with
1 cup rice flour, 2 teaspoons baking powder, and ½ teaspoon sea salt.

1. Preheat the oven to 400°F.

2. Place the baking mix in a large mixing bowl and set side. To a blender, add the egg, milk, oil, stevia, and corn, and blend well. Pour this mixture into the baking mix and stir until just mixed. Do not overstir.

3. Spoon the batter into a lightly oiled or papered mini muffin tin. Fill each cup with a heaping tablespoon of batter and bake for about 12 minutes. When a toothpick inserted into the center of a muffin comes out clean, the muffins are done.

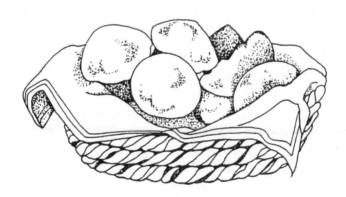

SWEET BUTTER BISCUITS

These biscuits are a delicious breakfast treat, either plain or topped with your favorite fruit spread. And if you like strawberry shortcake, these sweet butter biscuits can serve as the perfect base.

Yield: 24 biscuits (1½ inch)

1¾ cups all-purpose flour
1 tablespoon double-acting baking powder
½ teaspoon sea salt
⅛ teaspoon white stevia powder
4 tablespoons chilled salted butter
¾ cup cream or milk

1. Preheat the oven to 325°F.

2. Sift together the flour, baking powder, salt, and stevia powder in a large mixing bowl.

3. Cut the butter into the dry ingredients with a pastry blender or two knives (used scissor fashion) until the mixture is crumbly.

4. Add the cream, and mix the ingredients with a wooden spoon to form a soft, tacky (not wet) dough.

5. Turn out the dough onto a lightly floured surface and knead about ten times.

6. Gently roll out the dough from the center to a ¾-inch thickness.

7. With a floured 1½-inch biscuit cutter, cut straight down into the dough. Place the rounds on an ungreased cookie sheet and bake 10 to 12 minutes, or until golden brown.

BREAKFAST AMBROSIA

Yield: 4 servings

6 large oranges
2 cups unsweetened dried or freshly grated coconut*
½ cup coarsely chopped pecans, almonds, or walnuts
¼ cup fresh orange juice
⅛ teaspoon white stevia powder, or to taste

* If using fresh coconut, make a hole in the shell with a clean ice pick or screw-driver and drain the milk. Place the drained coconut in a preheated 400°F oven, and bake for about 15 minutes. While the shell is still hot, crack it open with a hammer. The meat should come out easily and cleanly. If it does not, pry it from the shell with a small heavy knife, and remove any brown skin with a vegetable peeler.

1. Peel the oranges, cutting away the white pith. Carefully separate the sections and remove the seeds

2. Place the orange sections, coconut, and nuts in a medium-sized mixing bowl and set aside.

3. Combine the orange juice and stevia, then pour it over the orange and nut mixture. Toss well. Cover with plastic wrap and chill in refrigerator for at least one hour before serving.

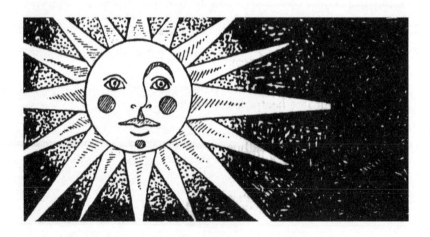

SALADS

and

DRESSINGS

Ginger Sweet Cole Slaw

Yield: 4 to 6 servings

SLAW

$1/2$ medium red cabbage, finely shredded
1 large red bell pepper, thinly sliced
$1/2$ medium red onion, thinly sliced

DRESSING

$1/3$ cup apple cider vinegar
3 tablespoons extra-virgin olive oil
1 tablespoon tamari, or other soy sauce
$1/2$ teaspoon finely chopped fresh ginger
$1/2$ teaspoon sea salt
$1/2$ teaspoon ground cardamom
$1/8$ teaspoon white stevia powder
Sesame seeds for garnish

1. Combine all of the dressing ingredients, except the sesame seeds, in a bowl or glass jar and mix well.

2. To prepare the slaw, place the cabbage, bell pepper, and onion in a salad bowl and mix well.

3. Pour the dressing evenly over the slaw and toss well.

4. Cover the bowl and chill in the refrigerator for several hours.

5. Garnish with sesame seeds before serving.

HOT-AND-SOUR CUCUMBER SALAD

Yield: 4 servings

1 pound cucumbers
1 teaspoon finely chopped garlic
½ fresh red chili pepper, finely sliced
1 teaspoon sea salt
¼ cup apple cider vinegar
2 to 4 drops stevia liquid concentrate, or to taste

1. Cut the cucumbers in half lengthwise, remove the seeds, then cut the halves into 3-inch slices.

2. Place the cucumbers in a salad bowl along with the remaining ingredients. Toss well, cover, and chill in the refrigerator for several hours. Occasionally stir the ingredients.

3. Drain thoroughly before serving.

CHILLED CUCUMBER SALAD

This dish is best when it has had time to marinate.
For best results, serve it the day after you've made it.

Yield: 4 servings

3 medium cucumbers
½ medium white onion, thinly sliced
2 stalks celery, thinly sliced diagonally

DRESSING
3 tablespoons apple cider vinegar
3 tablespoons tamari, or other soy sauce
1 tablespoon Dijon-style mustard

1 tablespoon freshly grated ginger
½ teaspoon coriander
⅛ teaspoon white stevia powder

1. Peel the cucumbers, quarter them lengthwise, and thinly slice. Place them in a salad bowl along with the onion and celery.

2. Combine all of the dressing ingredients in a small bowl or glass jar and mix well. Add the dressing to the vegetables and toss well.

3. Cover the bowl and chill in the refrigerator for at least 2 hours before serving.

GREEN AND WHITE JADE SALAD

Yield: 4 servings

8 ounces broccoli, cut into small florets
8 ounces cauliflower, cut into small florets
1 teaspoon sea salt

DRESSING
2 tablespoons tahini*
1 tablespoon apple cider vinegar
1 tablespoon tamari, or other soy sauce
1 teaspoon chili oil
1 teaspoon toasted sesame oil
1 teaspoon sea salt
4 drops stevia liquid concentrate, or to taste

* Tahini, or sesame seed paste, is available in most grocery stores.

1. Bring a medium-sized pot of water to boil. Add the broccoli, cauliflower, and salt. Blanch the vegetables for about 4 minutes, or until the broccoli turns bright green and is somewhat crisp yet tender.

2. Plunge the broccoli and cauliflower into cold water to prevent further cooking, then drain well in a colander. Arrange the vegetables on a platter.

3. Combine all of the dressing ingredients in a small bowl or glass jar and mix well. Pour the dressing over the vegetables and serve.

WALDORF SALAD

Yield: 4 to 6 servings

7 to 8 red Delicious apples, unpeeled, cored,
and cut into ½-inch cubes (about 4 cups)
1 cup raisins
1 cup coarsely chopped pecans
1 cup shredded carrot
¼ cup plus 2 tablespoons shredded unsweetened coconut

DRESSING
1-x-1-inch piece fresh ginger
1 cup mayonnaise
½ cup lemon juice
⅛ teaspoon white stevia powder

1. Grate the ginger. Using your hands, squeeze its juice into a small bowl. Add the mayonnaise, lemon juice, and stevia. Mix well.

2. In a salad bowl, combine the apples, raisins, pecans, carrot, and coconut. Add the dressing and toss well.

3. Cover the bowl and chill in the refrigerator for several hours before serving.

FRUIT RING SALAD

Yield: 6 to 8 servings
---

1 cup fresh orange juice
3 heaping tablespoons agar flakes*
1 teaspoon white stevia powder
1 cup kefir,** or buttermilk
1 cup sliced ripe strawberries
2 large peaches, peeled and thinly sliced
Fresh salad greens for garnish

* Available in health food stores, agar—also known as kanten—is a natural gelling agent.

** A cultured, enzyme-rich beverage, kefir contains friendly bacteria and beneficial yeast that help balance the body's "inner ecosystem." It supplies complete protein, essential minerals, and valuable B vitamins. Kefir is sold in health food stores or it can be made at home from a starter.

1. Place the orange juice, agar flakes, and stevia powder in a small saucepan and simmer over medium-low heat, stirring occasionally until the agar is completely dissolved.

2. Transfer the liquid to a large mixing bowl, and stir in the kefir. Add all of the remaining ingredients and mix well.

3. Spoon the mixture into a medium ring mold that has just been dipped into cold water. Place the mold in the refrigerator and chill for several hours, or until firm.

4. When the mold is set, line a round serving plate with salad greens, then place the unmolded ring on top. Slice and serve.

COOL HIJIKI SUMMER SLAW

Yield: 8 servings

SLAW
$\frac{1}{2}$ cup dried hijiki
$\frac{1}{2}$ medium green cabbage
$\frac{1}{2}$ medium red cabbage
1 medium cucumber, peeled and thinly sliced
1 medium red bell pepper, thinly sliced
1 tablespoon Herbamare, or sea salt
1 tablespoon organic, unrefined sesame oil
2 teaspoons tamari, or other soy sauce
1 teaspoon sea salt
$\frac{1}{4}$ cup sesame seeds for garnish (optional)

DRESSING
$\frac{1}{2}$ cup apple cider vinegar
$\frac{1}{2}$ cup Garlic-Chili-Flaxseed Oil Dressing (page 80)
2 teaspoons grated lemon rind
$\frac{1}{2}$ teaspoon ground coriander
$\frac{1}{8}$ teaspoon white stevia powder

1. Soak the hijiki in cold water for 15 to 20 minutes. Squeeze out the excess water and coarsely chop.

2. While the hijiki is soaking, finely grate the cabbage in a food processor.

3. Combine the cabbage, hijiki, cucumber, bell pepper, Herbamare, sesame oil, tamari, and salt in a large bowl and toss well.

4. Combine all of the dressing ingredients in a small bowl or jar and mix together. Pour the dressing over the slaw and toss well.

5. Cover the bowl and chill in the refrigerator for several hours.

6. Garnish with sesame seeds, if desired, before serving.

TARRAGON POTATO SALAD

Yield: 8 cups

6 cups cooked, diced red-skin potatoes (unpeeled)
2 cups frozen peas, thawed
1 cup finely diced red onion
1 large red bell pepper, finely diced
1 tablespoon sea salt

SWEET TARRAGON MAYONNAISE
2 egg yolks
2 tablespoons apple cider vinegar
1 tablespoon fresh lemon juice
$\frac{1}{2}$ teaspoon mustard
1 teaspoon sea salt
4 drops stevia liquid concentrate
1 tablespoon tarragon herb salad seasoning*
1 cup olive oil

* Spice Hunter brand is recommended.

1. Place the potatoes, peas, onion, and bell pepper in a large bowl, sprinkle with salt, and toss well. Set aside.

2. Place all of the mayonnaise ingredients and $\frac{1}{4}$ cup of the oil in a blender and blend for 30 seconds. With the blender still running, slowly add the remaining oil through the opening in the lid. Continue to blend until smooth.

3. Add $\frac{1}{4}$ cup of the mayonnaise to the potato salad ingredients and mix well. Add additional dressing as desired. Cover the salad and place in the refrigerator for at least 1 hour before serving. If there is any remaining mayonnaise, place it in a jar or container with a tight-fitting lid and refrigerate. It will keep for up to 2 weeks.

GARLIC-CHILI-FLAXSEED OIL DRESSING

Yield: 3 cups

1½ cups water
½ cup lemon juice
¼ cup garlic-and-chili-flavored flaxseed oil*
¼ cup organic, unrefined sesame oil
¼ cup apple cider vinegar
4 teaspoons finely chopped garlic
1 teaspoon tamari, or other soy sauce
2 drops stevia liquid concentrate (as a flavor enhancer)
1 teaspoon sea salt
½ teaspoon xanthan gum**

* Omega Nutrition Garlic-Chili Flaxseed Oil is recommended; however, you can substitute this ingredient with ¼ cup plain flaxseed oil, 1 clove chopped fresh garlic, and ⅛ teaspoon cayenne pepper.

** A natural, gluten-free carbohydrate commonly used as a thickener, xanthan gum is available in health food stores.

1. Place all of the ingredients, except the xanthan gum, in a blender, and blend thoroughly.

2. Add the xanthan gum, continuing to blend until the mixture has thickened.

3. Use immediately, or store in a tightly sealed container in the refrigerator. It will keep for up to two weeks.

JOHNNY'S FRENCH DRESSING

Cooking the tomatoes really concentrates their flavor; adding the flaxseed oil further enhances their taste.

Yield: 3 cups

4 plum tomatoes

1 teaspoon extra-virgin olive oil

1 teaspoon sea salt

1 cup apple cider vinegar

1 cup water

$\frac{1}{4}$ cup unrefined, organic safflower oil

$\frac{1}{4}$ cup flaxseed oil

2 teaspoons lecithin granules*

1 teaspoon tarragon

$\frac{1}{2}$ teaspoon Herbamare, or sea salt

$\frac{1}{8}$ teaspoon white stevia powder

$\frac{1}{4}$ teaspoon xanthan gum**

* Readily available in health food stores, lecithin is a flavorful, nutrient-rich binding agent that adds a creamy quality to products.

** A natural, gluten-free carbohydrate commonly used as a thickener, xanthan gum is available in health food stores.

1. Cut the tomatoes into quarters and remove the seeds. Set aside.

2. Preheat the olive oil in a 2-quart pot over medium-low heat. Add the tomatoes and salt, and sauté for 3 to 4 minutes, or until soft.

3. Add the apple cider vinegar and simmer until the mixture is about $\frac{1}{3}$ reduced. Transfer the mixture to a large mixing bowl and allow to cool to room temperature.

4. Add the remaining ingredients (except the xanthan gum). Using a hand-held mixer, blend the ingredients thoroughly at low speed.

5. Add the xanthan gum, and blend until the mixture thickens.

6. Transfer the mixture to a tightly sealed container and chill in the refrigerator until ready to serve. It will keep for up to 1 week.

SHALLOT AND POPPY SEED DRESSING

Yield: 2 cups

2 cups water
¾ cup finely chopped shallots
½ cup apple cider vinegar
¼ cup lemon juice
2 tablespoons lecithin granules*
2 teaspoons poppy seeds
2 teaspoons sea salt
¼ teaspoon white stevia powder
½ teaspoon xanthan gum**

* Readily available in health food stores, lecithin is a flavorful, nutrient-rich binding agent that adds a creamy quality to products.

** A natural, gluten-free carbohydrate commonly used as a thickener, xanthan gum is available in health food stores.

1. Combine all of the ingredients, except the xanthan gum, in a blender, and blend thoroughly.

2. Add the xanthan gum, continuing to blend until the mixture has thickened.

3. Use immediately, or store in a tightly sealed container in the refrigerator. It will keep for up to 1 week.

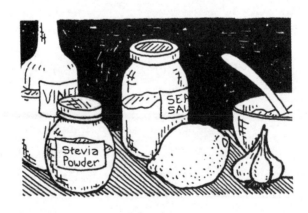

JAPANESE-STYLE DRESSING

Yield: 1½ cups

1 cup rice vinegar
¼ cup water
3 tablespoons tamari, or other soy sauce
2 tablespoons toasted sesame oil
1 tablespoon sea salt
2 to 4 drops stevia liquid concentrate

1. Place all of the ingredients in a small bowl or jar and mix well.

2. Cover and chill in the refrigerator for several hours before serving.

MISO MUSTARD DRESSING

Yield: ⅔ cup

2 tablespoons sweet white miso, or light barley miso
1 teaspoon Dijon-style mustard
2 tablespoons plus 1 teaspoon apple cider vinegar
6 drops stevia liquid concentrate
½ cup extra-virgin olive oil

1. In a small mixing bowl, combine the miso, mustard, vinegar, and stevia. Mash the ingredients together until well combined.

2. While slowly adding the oil, begin blending the mixture with a whisk or an electric hand-held mixer for 2 to 3 minutes, or until the oil is well blended with the ingredients. Transfer the dressing to a small jar with a lid and shake well. Use immediately, or store in the refrigerator for several days.

TARRAGON AND FENNEL DRESSING

Yield: 2 cups

2 cups water
½ cup apple cider vinegar, or freshly squeezed lemon juice
½ cup finely chopped fennel stalks
¼ cup fresh tarragon leaves, or 1 tablespoon dried
½ teaspoon sea salt
½ teaspoon white stevia powder
½ teaspoon xanthan gum*

* A natural, gluten-free carbohydrate commonly used as a thickener, xanthan gum is available in health food stores.

1. Place all of the ingredients except the xanthan gum in a blender, and blend thoroughly.

2. Add the xanthan gum, and blend until the mixture has thickened.

3. Transfer the mixture to a tightly sealed container and chill in the refrigerator until ready to serve. It will keep for up to 4 days.

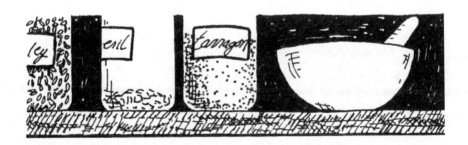

SATISFYING ENTRÉES and SIDE DISHES

SWEET VEGETARIAN CHILI

Yield: 8 servings

2 tablespoons extra-virgin olive oil
2 medium onions, coarsely diced
3 cloves garlic, finely chopped
4 medium green bell peppers, diced into 1-inch pieces
2 cups coarsely diced carrots
4 cups coarsely diced yellow squash
10 cups water
4 cups canned pinto beans
6-ounce can tomato paste
½ cup apple cider vinegar
1 jalapeño pepper, finely chopped
3 tablespoons Herbamare, or sea salt
2 tablespoons paprika
2 teaspoons chili powder
1 teaspoon dried oregano
¼ teaspoon white stevia powder

1. Place the olive oil in a 4-quart pot and preheat over medium-low heat. Add the onions and garlic, and sauté for 2 to 3 minutes, or until the onions are translucent and the garlic is lightly brown.

2. Add the bell peppers, carrots, and squash to the pot, and continue to sauté for 5 to 10 minutes.

3. Stir in the remaining ingredients. Simmer covered, stirring frequently, for about 2 hours, or until the liquid is somewhat reduced and the chili is thick.

4. Spoon the hot chili into bowls and serve.

CURRY CHICKEN

Yield: 8 servings

8 boneless, skinless chicken breasts,
cut into bite-sized pieces
2 cups flour
2 tablespoons salted butter
4 cups hot, cooked rice
Chopped scallions for garnish

CURRY SAUCE
⅓ cup salted butter
½ cup finely chopped onion
1 tablespoon curry powder
⅛ teaspoon white stevia powder
1 teaspoon sea salt
¼ teaspoon ginger
⅓ cup wheat flour
2 cups milk
2 cups chicken broth
1 teaspoon lemon juice

1. To make the sauce, melt the butter in a 2-quart pot over low heat (be careful not to burn it). Add the onion and sauté about 5 minutes, or until translucent. Gradually stir in the curry powder, stevia, salt, ginger, and flour, and mix well. Continue to cook, stirring frequently, until smooth.

2. While stirring constantly, slowly add the milk, broth, and lemon juice. Increase the heat to medium, and bring the sauce to a gentle boil while continuing to stir. Remove from the heat and cover to keep warm.

3. Lightly coat the chicken pieces in the flour. In a large nonstick skillet, melt the butter over medium-low heat. Add the chicken pieces and sauté until browned and no longer pink in the middle.

5. Place the hot rice on a serving platter, and top with the chicken. Spoon the curry sauce over the chicken, garnish with chopped scallions, and serve.

Variation

You can substitute the chicken with shrimp, beef, or your favorite vegetables.

SPINACH AND RICE NOODLES

Yield: 2 to 3 servings

4 ounces rice noodles
1 tablespoon tamari, or other soy sauce
2 teaspoons chili oil
2 to 3 drops stevia liquid concentrate
1 tablespoon sesame oil
2 tablespoons coarsely chopped garlic
1 teaspoon sea salt
1½ pounds fresh spinach, thoroughly washed and stemmed

1. Soak the rice noodles in a bowl of warm water for 25 minutes. Drain well and set aside.

2. Place the soy sauce, chili oil, and stevia in a cup, and stir well. Set aside.

3. Heat the sesame oil in a wok or large, deep skillet over medium heat. Add the garlic and salt, and stir-fry for a few seconds. Toss the spinach leaves into the wok and stir-fry for 2 minutes.

4. When the spinach is about two-thirds reduced, add the rice noodles and stevia mixture. Continue to stir-fry for another 4 minutes, or until the noodles are heated through.

5. Transfer the spinach and noodles to a serving bowl. Enjoy hot or cold.

CHOPPED CHICKEN SALAD

Yield: 4 servings

---

4 cups cooked chicken, chopped into bite-sized pieces
1 cup finely chopped red onion
1 cup finely chopped celery
1 cup finely chopped red bell pepper
1 teaspoon sea salt

VINAIGRETTE

$\frac{1}{2}$ cup raw, organic apple cider vinegar
$\frac{1}{2}$ cup freshly squeezed lemon juice
1 cup olive oil
4 tablespoons Dijon-style mustard
1 teaspoon freshly ground black pepper
1 teaspoon dried rosemary
$\frac{1}{2}$ teaspoon sea salt
4 to 6 drops stevia liquid concentrate
1 teaspoon xanthan gum (optional)*

* A natural, gluten-free carbohydrate commonly used as a thickener, xanthan gum is available in health food stores.

1. Place all of the vinaigrette ingredients, except the xanthan gum, in a small bowl and whisk together until well blended. Slowly add the xanthan gum, if using, while stirring constantly. Set aside.

2. Place the chicken, onion, celery, bell pepper, and salt in a medium-sized bowl. Add the vinaigrette and toss the ingredients together well. Cover and refrigerate several hours to allow the salad to marinate.

3. Serve chilled over a bed of mixed field greens.

TURKEY BURGERS WITH SWEET MUSTARD SAUCE

Yield: 4 burgers

BURGERS

1 pound ground turkey
2 teaspoons sea salt
1 tablespoon coconut oil or salted butter

MUSTARD SAUCE

4 tablespoons Dijon-style mustard
1 teaspoon dry mustard
8 to 10 drops stevia liquid concentrate
2 tablespoons apple cider vinegar
$^1/_2$ cup olive oil
$^1/_2$ cup chopped fresh dill, or 1 teaspoon dried

1. To make the mustard sauce, whisk the mustard, dry mustard, stevia, and vinegar together in a medium-sized bowl. Slowly add the oil, continuing to whisk the mixture until it is thick and well blended. Stir in the dill. Cover and refrigerate at least 1 hour.

2. Place the turkey and salt in a medium-sized bowl and mix well. Divide the mixture into four equal-sized patties.

3. Heat the coconut oil in a large skillet over medium heat. Add the patties and cook for 5 to 7 minutes. Turn the burgers over and continue to cook another 5 minutes, or until they are no longer pink inside when cut with a knife.

4. Serve the burgers hot, topped with sweet mustard sauce.

Sweet-and-Sour Tempeh

Yield: 4 servings

2 packages tempeh (8 ounces each), cut into $\frac{1}{2}$-inch cubes*
2 tablespoons olive oil, coconut oil, or butter
$1\frac{1}{2}$ large onions, diced
2 stalks celery, thinly sliced
1 large red bell pepper, coarsely diced
$1\frac{1}{2}$ cups water
1 teaspoon sea salt
4 cups cooked basmati rice

MARINADE
$\frac{1}{4}$ cup tamari, or other soy sauce
2 tablespoons apple cider vinegar
2 tablespoons water
$\frac{1}{8}$ teaspoon stevia liquid concentrate, or to taste
4 cloves garlic, minced

* Lightlife brand organic garden veggie or soy tempeh is recommended.

1. Combine the marinade ingredients in a small bowl or a 2-quart jar with a lid. If using a bowl, transfer the marinade to a gallon-size resealable baggie. Add the tempeh to the jar or baggie, seal, and shake well to coat the tempeh. Allow the tempeh to marinate at least 20 minutes and preferably over an hour. (The longer the tempeh marinates, the better it will be.)

2. Heat the oil in a large skillet or wok over medium heat. Add the onions and sauté 3 to 4 minutes, or until translucent. Add the celery and bell pepper, and sauté another 5 minutes, or until soft.

3. Add the tempeh and marinade to the skillet, and stir well with the other ingredients. Simmer uncovered for 10 minutes.

4. Stir in the water and salt, cover, and reduce the heat to medium-low. Simmer for about 20 minutes. If increased sweetness is desired, add additional drops of stevia.

5. Serve hot over basmati rice.

Variation

Try serving this dish chilled over a bed of green leaf lettuce.

RICE NOODLES WITH VEGETABLES

Yield: 2 to 3 servings

2 tablespoons coconut oil or salted butter
1 ounce fresh shiitake mushrooms
1/2 cup finely shredded carrots
1 small onion, finely diced
1/2 cup water
4 ounces bean thread noodles

SAUCE

1/4 cup tamari, or other soy sauce
3 tablespoons sesame oil
1 1/2 tablespoons sesame seeds
1 tablespoon finely chopped garlic
4 drops stevia liquid concentrate
1 teaspoon freshly ground black pepper

1. Heat the coconut oil in a wok or large deep skillet over medium heat. Add the mushrooms, carrots, onion, and water. Stir-fry for 5 minutes, or until the carrots are tender.

2. Combine all of the sauce ingredients and add them to the wok. Toss the ingredients well, then add the noodles. Stir-fry for 2 minutes, or until the mixture is thoroughly heated.

3. Serve hot or at room temperature.

SWEET-'N-SOUR VEGETABLE STIR-FRY

Yield: 4 servings

1 teaspoon sesame oil
4 cups thinly sliced red onion
5 to 6 cloves garlic, crushed
1 cup finely diced red bell pepper
1 tablespoon thinly sliced ginger
2 drops stevia liquid concentrate
2 teaspoons sea salt, or Herbamare
½ medium white cabbage, shredded
½ medium red cabbage, shredded
2 cups shredded carrots
2 cups cooked basmati rice
½ cup Teriyaki Sweet-'n-Sour Sauce (page 102)
6 to 8 chopped fresh mint leaves

1. Heat the oil in a wok or large deep skillet over medium heat. Add the onion, garlic, bell pepper, ginger, stevia, and salt, and stir-fry for 3 to 4 minutes, or until the onion and bell pepper are just beginning to soften.

2. Toss the cabbage and carrots into the wok, and continue to cook for 4 to 5 minutes, or until the cabbage and carrots are soft and wilted.

3. Add the rice and sweet-'n-sour sauce to the wok, and toss all of the ingredients together until they are well combined and heated through.

4. Add the mint leaves, and toss lightly before serving.

SWEET-'N-SOUR SAVORY CABBAGE

Yield: 4 to 6 servings

1 small head green cabbage
1 small head red cabbage
1 medium Vidalia onion, thinly sliced
$\frac{1}{2}$ cup apple cider vinegar
$\frac{1}{4}$ teaspoon white stevia powder
1 tablespoon salted butter
1 teaspoon coriander
$\frac{1}{2}$ teaspoon cardamom

1. Peel off and discard the outer leaves from the cabbage. Cut the heads in half, remove the core, and cut the cabbage into $\frac{1}{4}$-inch-thick slices.

2. Combine the vinegar and stevia in a small bowl and stir well. Set aside.

3. Heat the butter in a 4-quart pot over medium heat. Add the onion and sauté for 3 to 4 minutes, or until translucent and beginning to brown. Add the cabbage and toss well with the onion.

4. Add the stevia mixture to the pot along with the coriander and cardamom, and mix the ingredients well. Reduce the heat to medium low, cover the pot, and continue to cook, stirring frequently, for 4 to 5 minutes, or until the cabbage is soft and fragrant.

5. Transfer the cabbage to a serving bowl and enjoy hot.

SWEET CREAM CORN

Yield: 4 to 6 servings

6 large ears sweet corn
2 tablespoons salted butter
1 medium white onion, diced
1-x-1-inch piece fresh ginger, thinly sliced
⅛ teaspoon white stevia powder
Dash nutmeg
1 cup whole milk
1 cup cream

1. Using a sharp knife, carefully remove the corn from the cob and set aside.

2. Heat the butter in a 4-quart pot over medium-low heat. Add the onion, and sauté for 3 to 4 minutes, or until soft and translucent. Add the corn, ginger, stevia, and nutmeg, and sauté for about 5 minutes, while stirring occasionally.

3. Stir in the milk and cream, and simmer gently for 5 to 6 minutes, or until the liquid is reduced by half. Stir occasionally.

4. Transfer the creamed corn to a serving bowl and enjoy immediately.

CINNAMON CARROTS

Yield: 4 servings

1 teaspoon coconut oil, or salted butter
1 medium red onion, thinly sliced
4 to 6 large carrots, sliced lengthwise into julienned strips
4 to 6 drops stevia liquid concentrate, or to taste
1 teaspoon cinnamon

1. Heat the oil in a large skillet over medium heat. Add the onion and sauté 3 to 4 minutes, or until soft and translucent.

2. Add the carrots and stevia to the skillet, sprinkle with cinnamon, and toss well.

3. Reduce the heat to very low, cover, and cook for about 20 to 30 minutes, or until the carrots are tender. Serve hot.

SWEET SPAGHETTI SQUASH

Yield: 4 servings

1 medium spaghetti squash
$\frac{1}{4}$ cup fresh lemon juice
$1\frac{1}{2}$ teaspoons liquid stevia concentrate

1. Preheat the oven to 400°F. Pierce the squash with a fork in several places, and place it whole on a baking sheet. Bake for 1 to $1\frac{1}{2}$ hours, or until soft

2. After removing the squash from the oven, slice it in half and remove the seeds. Using a fork, remove the squash gently from its shell and place it in a bowl. The squash will be stringy, like spaghetti.* Add the lemon juice and stevia, and mix well.

3. Serve hot, at room temperature, or chilled.

* If the squash does not pull away from the shell easily, it is undercooked. Mushy squash indicates that it is overcooked.

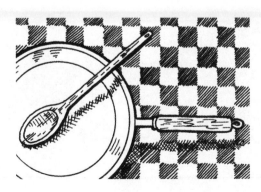

ASPARAGUS AND SUMMER SQUASH MEDLEY

Yield: 4 servings

2 cups asparagus tips (2-inch pieces)
1 tablespoon salted butter
1 cup diced red onion
4 cups coarsely diced yellow summer squash
2 to 4 drops stevia liquid concentrate
Sea salt to taste
⅓ cup coarsely chopped mint leaves

1. Bring a 2-quart pot of water to boil and add the asparagus; blanch for 2 to 3 minutes, or until tender yet crisp. Plunge the blanched asparagus into cold water, then drain well, and set aside.

2. Heat the butter in a large skillet over medium-low heat. Add the onion and sauté for 3 to 4 minutes, or until soft and translucent.

3. Add the squash, stevia, and sea salt. Continue sautéing for 5 to 6 minutes, or until the squash becomes soft and tender.

4. Add the asparagus and mint leaves, and toss the ingredients well. Cover the skillet, remove from the heat, and let sit 5 to 7 minutes, or until the mint leaves have wilted. Stir once more before serving.

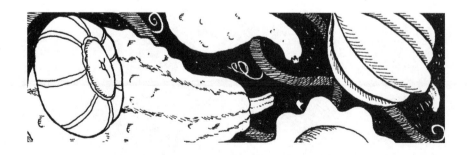

SAUCES, FROSTINGS, and OTHER TOPPINGS

SAVORY BLACKBERRY CHEESE SAUCE

*This delicious sauce is the perfect topping
for crepes, waffles, or pancakes.*

Yield: About 2 cups

1 tablespoon unsalted (sweet) butter
1 teaspoon chopped fresh garlic
¼ cup finely diced red onion
1 tablespoon grated lemon rind
¼ cup heavy cream
¼ teaspoon white stevia powder
*8-ounce package cream cheese or Neufchatel cheese,
at room temperature*
10-ounce package frozen blackberries, thawed, or 1 pint fresh

1. Melt the butter in a medium-sized nonstick skillet over medium heat. Add the garlic and sauté 1 to 2 minutes, or until beginning to soften.

2. Add the onions and lemon peel to the skillet, and continue to sauté another few minutes until the onions are translucent.

3. Reduce the heat to low, and stir in the cream and stevia. Simmer, stirring frequently, just until the ingredients are well blended. Remove from the heat and set aside.

4. Place the cream cheese in a medium-sized mixing bowl, and whip with a fork until soft and fluffy. Stir in the garlic-onion mixture until well-combined. Fold in the blackberries.

5. Use immediately, or store in the refrigerator up to four days.

Variation

For a sweeter, less savory sauce, simply eliminate the onions and garlic.

Teriyaki Sweet-'n-Sour Sauce

We suggest using this sauce in Sweet-'n-Sour Vegetable Stir-Fry (page 94), but feel free to use it to liven up any number of entrées and side dishes.

Yield: About 2¾ cups

1 teaspoon sesame oil
1 tablespoon finely chopped scallion
½-x-½-inch piece fresh ginger, thinly sliced
¼ cup chopped red bell pepper
2 tablespoons tamari, or other soy sauce
1 tablespoon apple cider vinegar
2 tablespoons organic tomato paste
⅛ teaspoon white stevia powder
⅛ teaspoon cayenne pepper
2 cups water, or vegetable or chicken stock
1 teaspoon cornstarch dissolved in ¼ cup water

1. Heat the oil in a stockpot over low heat. Add the scallion, ginger, and bell pepper, and sauté for 5 minutes, or until the peppers are just beginning to soften.

2. Add the soy sauce and vinegar, and simmer for about 3 to 4 minutes, or until the liquid is reduced by half.

3. Add the tomato paste, stevia, cayenne pepper, and water to the pot. Increase the heat to medium, and bring the ingredients to a light boil for 5 minutes.

6. Using a hand-held mixer, purée the ingredients until very smooth.

7. Add the cornstarch mixture to the pot, stir well, and bring to a boil. Reduce the heat to low and simmer for 15 minutes, stirring occasionally.

8. Use the sauce immediately, or transfer it to a tightly sealed container and store in the refrigerator where it will keep for up to four days.

MAPLE SYRUP

Yield: About ¾ cup

¾ cup filtered water
2 tablespoons plus 2 teaspoons vegetable glycerine*
2 teaspoons nonalcoholic maple flavoring
⅛ teaspoon white stevia powder

* Derived from coconut oil, vegetable glycerine is a sweet-tasting thickener. It is available in most health food stores.

1. Combine all of the ingredients in a small bowl and mix well. You can also place the ingredients in a clean glass jar, cover with a lid, and shake thoroughly.

2. Warm the mixture in a small pan before drizzling it over pancakes, waffles, or hot cereal.

SWEET WHIPPED CREAM

Yield: 2 cups

1 pint whipping cream
⅛ teaspoon white stevia powder

1. Place the cream in a large mixing bowl and beat with a whisk or an electric hand-held mixer until it begins to thicken.

2. Sprinkle the stevia over the cream and continue to beat until soft peaks form (do not overbeat).

3. Use immediately or place in an airtight container and refrigerate up to four days.

TANGELO THYME SAUCE

Enjoy this as a sauce for stir-fries, a glaze for poultry dishes, or a topping for ice cream or frozen yogurt.

Yield: 1½ cups

1 teaspoon salted butter
1 shallot, finely diced
Several sprigs coarsely chopped fresh thyme
Juice of 4 large tangelos (about 1½ cups)
2 teaspoons cornstarch, or arrowroot powder
4 drops stevia liquid concentrate

1. Heat the butter in a 2-quart pot over medium heat. Add the shallot and sauté for 2 to 3 minutes, or until translucent. Add the thyme and continue to sauté another minute.

2. Add the stevia and cornstarch to the tangelo juice and stir to dissolve. Pour this mixture into the pot, reduce the heat to low, and simmer, stirring frequently, for 10 to 15 minutes, or until the mixture thickens.

3. Use immediately, or place in a tightly sealed container and refrigerate for several days.

CAROB FUDGE SAUCE

*Delicious served over puddings, ice creams,
or whenever a carob sauce is desired.*

Yield: 1 cup

*8 ounces heavy cream
1¼ cups unsweetened carob chips
¼ teaspoon white stevia powder (or to taste)
1 teaspoon or more vanilla flavoring*

1. Place the cream in a 2-quart pot, and place over low heat.

2. Slowly add the carob chips and stevia powder, stirring frequently until chips begin to melt.

3. Remove from the heat and cool slightly. Stir in the vanilla flavoring.

4. Use immediately, or store in the refrigerator for several days.

Variation

For a chocolate sauce, substitute 1-ounce square unsweetened chocolate for the carob chips, and include enough stevia to achieve desired sweetness.

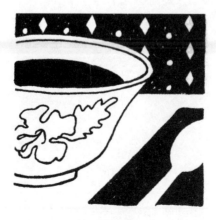

FAVORITE CHOCOLATE CREAM CHEESE FROSTING

Yield: Enough to frost two 9-inch single layer cakes,
1 dozen standard muffins, or 2 dozen mini muffins.

*2 packages (8 ounces each) cream cheese,
at room temperature*
$\frac{1}{2}$ teaspoon white stevia powder
3 tablespoons skim milk
$\frac{1}{3}$ cup organic cocoa powder
1 teaspoon vanilla flavoring

1. Place the cream cheese, stevia, and 1 tablespoon of the milk in a small bowl, and whisk until fluffy.

2. Stir in the cocoa, vanilla, and enough of the remaining milk to form a smooth, spreadable frosting.

3. Use immediately, or store in the refrigerator for several days.

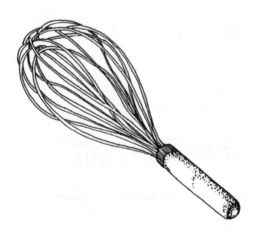

HEAVENLY

CAKES

and PIES

Some Reminders About Baking With Stevia

Remember, as detailed in "Cooking With Stevia," beginning on page 49, stevia is not perfect when it comes to baked goods. Baked items sweetened with stevia do not rise as well as those made with sugar, and because stevia does not aid in the fermentation of yeast, it is not a good sugar substitute for yeasted breads and cakes. Baked goods made with stevia do not brown as well as those made with sugar.

Although the cake and muffin recipes found in this chapter are sweetened with stevia only, know that you can opt to use it as a partial sugar replacement, if you prefer. (See Equivalency Chart on page 54.) This applies to any of your favorite recipes, as well as the ones found in this chapter. Replacing even half the sugar called for in a recipe with stevia will produce a fine product with less calories than those made solely with sugar.

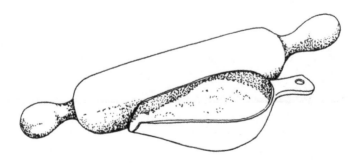

SPICY CARROT CAKE

Yield: 9-inch round, single-layer cake

2 cups all-purpose baking mix*
1 teaspoon guar gum (optional)
2 cups finely chopped or grated carrots
½ cup coarsely chopped raisins
½ cup shredded unsweetened coconut
2 eggs
1 cup heavy cream
¼ cup water
2 teaspoons ground cinnamon
1 teaspoon ground nutmeg
½ teaspoon ground ginger
½ teaspoon white stevia powder
½ cup chopped pecans

*Arrowhead Mills brand is recommended.

1. Preheat oven to 350°F. Butter and flour a 9-inch springform pan.

2. Sift together the baking mix and guar gum (if using) and set aside.

3. Place the carrots, raisins, and coconut in a blender, and pulse until finely ground. Add to the flour.

4. Beat the eggs with a fork or whisk until light and fluffy. Set aside.

5. Place the cream, water, cinnamon, nutmeg, ginger, and stevia in a small saucepan over low heat. Stir until the mixture is warm and aromatic. (Do not let it get too hot or the cream will curdle.)

6. Slowly add the cream mixture and eggs to the flour mixture, stirring until the batter is well combined.

7. Spoon the batter into the prepared cake pan and bake about 30 minutes, or until a toothpick inserted into the center comes out clean.

8. When the cake is cool enough to handle, carefully remove the sides of the springform pan. Serve warm or at room temperature.

CHOCOLATE AMARANTH TORTE

Yield: 9-inch round, single-layer cake

4 cups water
½ cup carob powder
2 cups amaranth, rinsed
2 cups cooked, mashed butternut squash
½ teaspoon white stevia powder

1. Lightly grease a 9-inch-round cake or springform pan, and set aside.

2. Place 1 cup of the water and the carob powder in a heavy 4-quart pot, and stir well to dissolve. Add the amaranth and the remaining water, and place over low heat. Cover and simmer, stirring occasionally, until the amaranth is tender and the mixture is thick.

3. Transfer the mixture to a large mixing bowl along with the squash and stevia. Using an electric hand-held mixer, blend the ingredients well. If necessary, add additional water to create a pudding-like consistency.*

5. Pour the mixture into the prepared pan, and refrigerate 1 to 2 hours or until firm.

6. Serve as is, or topped with a dollop of Sweet Whipped Cream (page 103).

* You can also use a blender or food processor for this step.

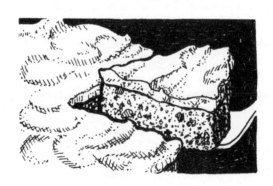

ALMOST FLOURLESS CHOCOLATE CAKE

This yummy chocolate cake is sugar-free.

Yield: 9-inch round, single-layer cake

$\frac{1}{4}$ *cup all-purpose flour*
$\frac{1}{8}$ *teaspoon sea salt*
6 tablespoons unsalted (sweet) butter
4 ounces unsweetened chocolate
$\frac{1}{3}$ *cup milk*
$\frac{1}{3}$ *cup apricot or raspberry 100% spreadable fruit*
2 teaspoons Dacopa, or other instant grain coffee substitute
1 teaspoon coffee flavoring (optional)
1 egg yolk, lightly beaten
1 tablespoon vanilla flavoring
1 teaspoon white stevia powder, or $\frac{1}{8}$ teaspoon liquid concentrate
3 egg whites
$\frac{1}{8}$ *teaspoon cream of tartar*

1. Preheat the oven to 350°F. Lightly grease the sides of a 9-inch round cake pan and line the bottom with parchment paper.

2. Combine the flour and sea salt in a small bowl and set aside.

3. Place the butter, chocolate, milk, fruit preserves, coffee substitute, and coffee flavoring (if using) in a small saucepan over medium-low heat. Stir constantly until the chocolate is almost melted. Remove the pan from the heat, and continue to stir until the chocolate is completely melted and the mixture is smooth.

4. Whisk the egg yolk and vanilla into the chocolate. Add the stevia and continue whisking until smooth. Set aside.

5. Using an electric hand-held mixer, beat the egg whites and cream of tartar until stiff peaks form. First fold the chocolate mixture into the egg whites to form a smooth batter, then fold the flour into the batter.

6. Pour the batter into the prepared pan and bake for 18 to 20 minutes, or until a toothpick inserted in the center comes out clean. Do not overbake.

7. Carefully loosen the cake from the sides of the pan with a small sharp knife. This will prevent the cake from cracking as it cools.

8. Allow the cake to cool completely in the pan, cover with wax paper, and place in the refrigerator for 1 to 2 hours to chill.

9. Remove the cake from the pan and cut into wedges. Serve as is, or topped with Sweet Whipped Cream (page 103) or one of your favorite preserves.

BANANA BUTTERNUT SQUASH CHEESECAKE

Yield: 9-inch round cake

4 cups cooked, mashed butternut squash
2 packages cream cheese (8 ounces each), at room temperature
3 ripe bananas
4 eggs
2 tablespoons vanilla flavoring
1 teaspoon ground spice blend*
¼ teaspoon white stevia powder

CRUST
1 cup finely crushed ginger snap cookies
4 tablespoons unsalted (sweet) butter, softened

* Spice Hunter Sweet Spice Blend is recommended.

1. Preheat the oven to 350°F. Butter a 9-inch springform cake pan, and set aside.

2. To make the crust, place the ginger snap crumbs and butter in a small bowl and mix until well combined. Using your hands, pat the mixture smoothly and evenly in the bottom of the pan.

3. Place the squash, cream cheese, bananas, eggs, vanilla, spice blend, and stevia in a large mixing bowl. Using an electric hand-held mixer, blend until smooth.

4. Pour the mixture into the prepared pan, then set the pan in a larger pan. Fill the larger pan with water—about $^3/_4$ the height of the cheesecake pan.

5. Place the pans on the center rack of the oven and bake for 1 hour, or until the cheesecake sets and the center of the cake is firm to the touch.

6. Remove the pans from the oven and place on a wire rack for 2 hours to cool completely. Once cool, remove the cheesecake pan from the water and refrigerate for 1 to 2 hours to chill.

7. Before removing the springform pan, loosen the cake from the sides with a knife.

8. Serve as is or topped with Sweet Whipped Cream (page 103).

BING CHERRY CHEESECAKE

Yield: 9-inch round cake

2 packages cream cheese (8 ounces each), at room temperature
4 eggs
$^1/_2$ cup lemon juice
2 tablespoons grated lemon rind
2 tablespoons vanilla flavoring
$^1/_2$ teaspoon cinnamon
$^1/_2$ teaspoon white stevia powder
3 cups finely chopped Bing cherries

CRUST
1 cup crushed graham crackers
4 tablespoons unsalted (sweet) butter, softened

1. Preheat the oven to 350°F. Butter a 9-inch springform cake pan, and set aside.

2. To make the crust, place the graham cracker crumbs and butter in a small bowl and mix until well combined. Using your hands, pat the mixture smoothly and evenly in the bottom of the pan. Set aside.

3. Place the cream cheese, eggs, lemon rind, vanilla, cinnamon, and stevia in a large mixing bowl. Using an electric hand-held mixer, blend until smooth. Fold in the cherries.

4. Pour the mixture into the prepared pan, then set the pan in a larger pan. Fill the larger pan with water—about $3/4$ the height of the cheesecake pan.

5. Place the pans on the center rack of the oven and bake for 30 to 40 minutes, or until the cheesecake sets and the center of the cake is firm to the touch.

6. Remove the pans from the oven and place on a wire rack for 2 hours to cool completely. Once cool, remove the cheesecake pan from the water and place it in the refrigerator for 1 to 2 hours to chill.

7. Before removing the springform pan, loosen the cake from the sides with a knife.

8. Serve as is or topped with a dollop of Sweet Whipped Cream (page 103).

BASIC PIE CRUST

Yield: Single 9-inch crust

1½ cups all-purpose flour
¼ teaspoon salt
⅛ teaspoon white stevia powder
4 tablespoons cold, unsalted (sweet) butter, thinly sliced
4 to 5 tablespoons ice cold water

1. Sift together the flour, salt, and stevia in a large mixing bowl.

2. Cut the butter into the flour using a pastry blender or two knives (used scissor style) until the mixture resembles coarse meal.

3. Sprinkle 1 tablespoon of water over the flour mixture, and toss lightly with a fork. Push the dampened mixture to the side of the bowl and continue sprinkling and tossing the dry portion with water. The dough should be just moist enough to hold together. (If the flour is wet and tacky, add a little more flour; if it is dry and crumbly, add a little more water.) Shape the mixture into a soft, pliable ball.

4. On a lightly floured surface, roll out the ball into an 11-inch circle. Fold the dough in half and transfer it to a 9-inch pie plate, making sure the fold is in the center. Unfold the dough and fit it carefully into the plate. Crimp the edges.

5. Fill the shell with the desired filling and bake as directed. For a pre-baked shell, prick the entire surface with a fork, and bake in a 350°F oven for 12 to 15 minutes, or until golden. Cool completely before filling.

SWEET GRAHAM CRACKER CRUST

Yield: Single 9-inch crust

1½ cups crushed graham crackers (about 20 crackers)
¼ cup shredded unsweetened coconut
4 tablespoons unsalted (sweet) butter, softened
⅛ teaspoon cinnamon
Scant ⅛ teaspoon white stevia powder, or 10 drops liquid concentrate

1. Combine all of the ingredients in a large mixing bowl.

2. Press the mixture on the bottom and sides of a 9-inch pie pan to form a smooth, even crust.

3. Fill the shell with the desired filling and bake as directed. For a prebaked shell, bake in a 375°F oven for about 8 minutes, or until golden. Cool completely before filling.

MOCHA CREAM PIE

Yield: 9-inch pie

2 cups heavy cream
¼ teaspoon white stevia powder
1¼ cups unsweetened carob chips
2 teaspoons Dacopa, or other instant grain coffee substitute
¾ cup water
1 level teaspoon agar flakes*
⅛ teaspoon white stevia powder
9-inch prebaked Basic Pie Crust (page 114),
or Sweet Graham Cracker Crust (page 115)
Toasted, shredded coconut for garnish

* Available in health food stores, agar—also known as kanten—is a natural jelling
agent.

1. Place 1 cup of the cream and ¼ teaspoon stevia in a 2-quart pot over medium heat. As the cream begins to warm, gradually add the carob chips and stir until they have melted.

2. Add the coffee substitute, water, and agar to the pot, and increase the temperature slightly. Stirring constantly, bring the mixture to a gentle simmer, and cook until it is smooth. Remove from the heat and let cool to room temperature.

3. Place the remaining cream and ⅛ teaspoon stevia in a large mixing bowl. Using an electric hand-held mixer, beat the mixture until soft peaks form. Do not overbeat.

4. Fold the cooled carob mixture into the whipped cream, blending carefully but thoroughly. Pour the filling mixture into the crust and refrigerate for at least 1 hour.

5. Before serving, garnish with toasted coconut.

SAVORY APPLE PIE

Yield: 9-inch pie

3 to 4 large Granny Smith apples
2 tablespoons fresh lemon juice
$\frac{1}{2}$ teaspoon cinnamon
$\frac{1}{8}$ teaspoon white stevia powder
2 tablespoons unsalted (sweet) butter
$\frac{1}{2}$ cup finely diced onion
$\frac{1}{2}$ cup crushed walnuts (or pecans)
$\frac{1}{2}$ cup kefir,* or buttermilk
1 tablespoon cornstarch dissolved in $\frac{1}{4}$ cup cold water
9-inch prebaked Basic Pie Crust (page 114)

* A cultured, enzyme-rich beverage, kefir contains friendly bacteria and beneficial yeast that help balance the body's "inner ecosystem." It supplies complete protein, essential minerals, and valuable B vitamins. Kefir is sold in health food stores, or it can be made at home from a starter.

1. Peel, core, and slice the apples, then place them in a large bowl. Sprinkle with lemon juice, cinnamon, and stevia, and toss well. Set aside.

2. Place the butter in a large skillet over medium heat. Add the onion and sauté about 10 minutes, or until golden brown and well caramelized.

3. Add the apples and nuts to the skillet, and continue to sauté for about 5 minutes, or until the apples are soft.

4. Stir the kefir and cornstarch mixture into the skillet, and continue to cook, stirring constantly, until the liquid thickens.

5. Pour the filling mixture into the crust and sprinkle with more crushed nuts. (If desired, you can pop the pie under the broiler for a minute to lightly toast the nuts.)

6. Serve hot or at room temperature.

PUMPKIN PIE

Yield: 9-inch pie

4 cups cooked, mashed butternut squash
1 teaspoon pumpkin spice
1 tablespoon vanilla flavoring
¼ teaspoon white stevia powder
Pinch sea salt
9-inch prebaked Basic Pie Crust (page 114)

1. Place all of the filling ingredients in a blender or food processor and blend until smooth and well-combined.

2. Pour the filling mixture into the crust and refrigerate for at least 1 hour.

3. Serve chilled or at room temperature, either plain or topped with a dollop of Sweet Whipped Cream (page 103).

BANANA COCONUT CREAM PIE

Yield: 9-inch pie

2 cups milk
4 egg yolks
¼ cup cornstarch
2 medium bananas, diced
½ cup toasted, shredded coconut
½ teaspoon vanilla flavoring
¼ teaspoon banana flavoring
¼ teaspoon white stevia powder
Pinch cinnamon
9-inch prebaked Basic Pie Crust (page 114)
Toasted, shredded coconut for garnish

1. Place the milk in a 2-quart pot and place over medium-high heat until the milk is scalded (just starting to come to a boil). Remove from the heat and allow the milk to cool to lukewarm.

2. Whisk the egg yolks and cornstarch together in a medium bowl until smooth. Drizzle the cooled milk very slowly into the egg mixture, stirring constantly, until well combined.

3. Return the mixture to the pot, place over medium heat, and stir constantly until the mixture begins to thicken slightly. Add the bananas, coconut, vanilla and banana flavorings, stevia, and cinnamon, and continue to cook until thickened.

4. Pour the filling mixture into the crust and garnish with toasted coconut. Refrigerate several hours.

5. Serve as is, or topped with a dollop of Sweet Whipped Cream (page 103).

LEMON CUSTARD PIE

Yield: 9-inch pie

4 egg yolks
¼ cup cornstarch
2 cups buttermilk
¾ cup lemon juice
Scant ¼ teaspoon white stevia powder
9-inch prebaked Basic Pie Crust (page 114)

1. Whisk the egg yolks and cornstarch together in a medium bowl until smooth. Add the buttermilk, lemon juice, and stevia, and mix well.

2. Transfer the mixture to a 2-quart pot and cook over medium-high heat, whisking constantly. Once the mixture thickens, reduce the heat to medium-low and continue to cook for another 2 minutes. The custard should be bubbling lightly at this point.

3. Pour the filling mixture into the crust, and refrigerate for 1 to 2 hours before serving.

VANILLA CAROB CUSTARD PIE

Yield: 9-inch pie

2 cups milk
4 egg yolks
¼ cup cornstarch
¾ teaspoon vanilla flavoring
⅛ teaspoon white stevia powder
¼ cup carob powder
9-inch prebaked Basic Pie Crust (page 114),
or Sweet Graham Cracker Crust (page 115)

1. Place the milk in a 2-quart pot and place over medium-high heat until the milk is scalded (just starting to come to a boil). Remove from the heat and allow the milk to cool to lukewarm.

2. Whisk the egg yolks and cornstarch together in a medium bowl until smooth. Add the vanilla and stevia, and mix well. Drizzle the cooled milk very slowly into the egg mixture, stirring constantly, until well combined.

3. Return the mixture to the pot, stir in the carob mixture, and place over medium heat. Stir constantly until the mixture is thick and smooth.

4. Pour the filling mixture into the crust, and refrigerate for 1 to 2 hours before serving.

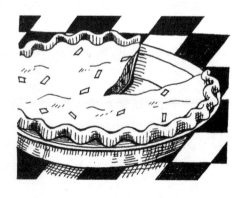

HOMESTYLE COOKIES, CANDY, and ICE CREAM

NORMA'S ALMOND BUTTER COOKIES

These delicious cookies are wheat-free.

Yield: About 2 dozen

$\frac{1}{2}$ cup unsalted (sweet) butter, softened
$\frac{3}{4}$ teaspoon white stevia powder
1 egg, lightly beaten
1 cup almond butter
2 teaspoons vanilla flavoring
$\frac{1}{2}$ teaspoon sea salt
$\frac{1}{2}$ teaspoon baking soda
$1\frac{1}{2}$ cups brown rice baking mix*

CINNAMON SPRINKLES
1 teaspoon ground cinnamon
$\frac{1}{8}$ teaspoon white stevia powder
Dash vanilla powder (optional)**

* Fern's brand is recommended; however, you can substitute this ingredient with $1\frac{1}{2}$ cups rice flour, 1 tablespoon baking powder, and $\frac{3}{4}$ teaspoon sea salt.

** Madagascar Bourbon Pure Vanilla Powder, which is available in many health food stores and gourmet shops, is recommended.

1. Preheat the oven to 350°F. Combine the cinnamon sprinkle ingredients in a small bowl and set aside. Lightly grease a cookie sheet.*

2. Place the butter in a medium-sized mixing bowl and whisk until light and fluffy. Stir the stevia into the beaten egg, then add it to the butter, along with the almond butter, vanilla, salt, and baking soda. Whisk until smooth.

3. Using a wooden spoon, add the rice flour, $\frac{1}{2}$ cup at a time, stirring well after each addition. The dough should be thick enough to hold its shape on a tablespoon.

4. Drop heaping teaspoons of cookie dough onto the cookie sheet, about 2 inches apart.

5. Lightly press each mound of dough with the back of a fork in a criss-cross pattern.

6. Sprinkle each cookie lightly with the cinnamon sprinkles, and bake 15 minutes, or until lightly browned.

* Instead of greasing a cookie sheet, you can cover it with parchment paper, which makes for quick and easy cleanup.

Variation

You can substitute peanut butter for almond butter and eliminate the cinnamon sprinkles.

CAROB ALMOND BUTTER CRISPIES

Yield: 2 dozen

1 cup almond butter
12 drops stevia liquid concentrate
3 heaping tablespoons ground flaxseed
2 tablespoons carob powder
2 tablespoons coconut oil, or butter
1 tablespoon vanilla flavoring
$\frac{1}{2}$ teaspoon sea salt
4 cups crushed crisped brown rice cereal
1 cup chopped pecans

1. Place the almond butter, stevia, flaxseed, carob, oil, vanilla, and salt in a large mixing bowl, and combine thoroughly. Stir in the crisped rice and pecans.

2. Shape the mixture into 2-inch balls, and serve.

Variation

For a more decorative candy, roll the balls in toasted coconut or more crushed rice crispies.

CHOCOLATE CHIP COOKIES

Yield: About 4 dozen

2 cups all-purpose flour
¾ teaspoon sea salt
¾ teaspoon baking powder
1 egg
½ teaspoon white stevia powder
1 teaspoon vanilla flavoring
1 cup salted butter, softened
1¼ cups chocolate chips

1. Preheat the oven to 350°F. Lightly grease a cookie sheet and set aside.*

2. In a medium mixing bowl, sift together the flour, salt, and baking powder, and set aside.

3. Place the egg, stevia, and vanilla in a large mixing bowl, and beat well with a wooden spoon or an electric hand-held mixer. Slowly add the butter, continuing to beat until the mixture is smooth and creamy.

4. Add the flour mixture to the butter mixture, ½ cup at a time, stirring well with a wooden spoon after each addition. Fold in the chocolate chips.

5. Drop heaping teaspoons of batter on the cookie sheet, about 2 inches apart. Bake for 20 to 25 minutes, or until the cookies are golden brown.

* Instead of greasing a cookie sheet, you can cover it with parchment paper, which makes for quick and easy cleanup.

COCONUT RAISIN QUINOA COOKIES

Yield: About 2 dozen
---

2 cups quinoa flakes
1 cup shredded unsweetened coconut
½ cup raisins
4 tablespoons unsalted (sweet) butter, softened
2 eggs
3 tablespoons water
2 tablespoons vanilla flavoring
¼ teaspoon cinnamon
¼ teaspoon coconut flavoring
¼ teaspoon white stevia powder
⅛ teaspoon pumpkin pie spice

1. Preheat the oven to 350°F. Lightly grease a cookie sheet and set aside.*

2. Combine all of the ingredients in a blender or food processor, and pulse until well combined and tacky.

3. Form the mixture into 2-inch balls, place about 2 inches apart on cookie sheet, and bake for 15 minutes, or until golden brown.

* Instead of greasing a cookie sheet, you can cover it with parchment paper, which makes for quick and easy cleanup.

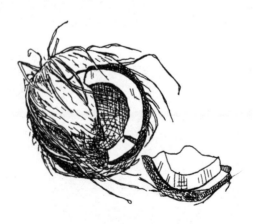

COCONUT MACAROONS

Yield: About 2 dozen

2 cups shredded unsweetened coconut
$\frac{1}{2}$ cup quinoa flakes
2 tablespoons salted butter, softened
2 teaspoons liquid lecithin*
$\frac{1}{8}$ teaspoon white stevia powder
4 egg whites
$\frac{1}{16}$ teaspoon white stevia powder

* Readily available in health food stores, lecithin is a flavorful, nutrient-rich binding agent that adds a creamy quality to products.

1. Preheat the oven to 350°F. Lightly grease a cookie sheet and set aside.*

2. Place the coconut, quinoa, lecithin, butter, and $\frac{1}{8}$ teaspoon stevia in a blender or food processor, and pulse until well combined. Transfer to a large mixing bowl.

3. Place the egg whites and $\frac{1}{16}$ teaspoon stevia in a medium mixing bowl, and beat with an electric hand-held mixer until stiff peaks form.

4. Fold the egg whites into the coconut mixture until thoroughly combined (you will lose most of the volume of the egg whites).

5. Form the mixture into 2-inch balls, place about 2 inches apart on cookie sheet, and bake for 10 minutes, or until golden brown.

* Instead of greasing a cookie sheet, you can cover it with parchment paper, which makes for quick and easy cleanup.

CURRANT OATMEAL COOKIES

Yield: About 2 dozen

$1\frac{1}{2}$ cups all-purpose flour
$\frac{1}{2}$ teaspoon sea salt
1 teaspoon baking powder
$\frac{1}{2}$ teaspoon grated nutmeg
1 cup unsalted (sweet) butter, softened
$\frac{3}{4}$ teaspoon white stevia powder
2 eggs
2 cups organic rolled oats
$1\frac{1}{4}$ cups currants

1. Preheat the oven to 350°F. Lightly grease a cookie sheet and set aside.*

2. In a medium mixing bowl, sift together the flour, salt, baking powder, and nutmeg, and set aside.

3. Place the butter in a large mixing bowl and whisk until light and fluffy. Add the stevia and eggs, one at a time, whisking well after each egg. Stir in the oats and currants.

4. Form the mixture into 2-inch balls, place about 2 inches apart on cookie sheet, and bake for 20 to 25 minutes, or until golden brown.

* Instead of greasing a cookie sheet, you can cover it with parchment paper, which makes for quick and easy cleanup.

Variations

- For cinnamon-raisin oatmeal cookies, simply substitute 1 cup raisins and $\frac{1}{4}$ teaspoon cinnamon for the currants and nutmeg.

- For chocolate oatmeal cookies, substitute $1\frac{1}{2}$ cups carob chips for the currants. For a low-sugar variation, use grain-sweetened chocolate chips or carob chips.

SWEET SUGARLESS COOKIES

Yield: About 1½ dozen

1½ cups all-purpose flour
½ teaspoon sea salt
½ teaspoon baking powder
¼ teaspoon grated nutmeg
2 eggs
½ teaspoon white stevia powder
1 cup unsalted (sweet) butter, softened

1. Preheat the oven to 350°F. Lightly grease a cookie sheet and set aside.*

2. In a medium mixing bowl, sift together the flour, salt, baking powder, and nutmeg, and set aside.

3. Place the eggs and stevia in a large bowl, and beat with an electric hand-held mixer until well combined. Slowly add the butter, continuing to beat until the mixture is smooth and creamy.

4. Using a wooden spoon, add the flour mixture to the butter mixture, ½ cup at a time, stirring well after each addition.

5. Form the dough into 2-inch balls and place them 2-inches apart on the cookie sheet. Flatten the balls slightly with the bottom of a glass. Bake for 20 to 25 minutes, or until the cookies are golden brown.

* Instead of greasing a cookie sheet, you can cover it with parchment paper, which makes for quick and easy cleanup.

Variations

- Place a pecan half on top of each cookie before baking.

- Flatten the balls slightly with the bottom of a juice glass, then make a thumblike depression in the center. Fill the depression with your favorite jelly, jam, chocolate chips, or carob chips before baking.

SHEREE'S LOW-SUGAR COOKIES

This original recipe called for 1 cup of sugar.

Yield: About 2 dozen

2 cups brown rice baking mix*
½ teaspoon baking soda
¼ teaspoon sea salt
1 cup unsalted (sweet) butter, softened
½ cup granulated sugar
¼ teaspoon stevia liquid concentrate
2 eggs
½ teaspoon vanilla flavoring

* Fern's brand is recommended; however, you can substitute this ingredient with 2 cups rice flour, 4 teaspoons baking powder, and 1 teaspoon sea salt.

1. Sift together the rice mix, baking soda, and salt in a medium bowl, and set aside.

2. Place the butter in a large mixing bowl and whisk until light and fluffy. Stir in the sugar and stevia. Add the eggs and vanilla, and continue to whisk until smooth.

3. Using a wooden spoon, stir the flour mixture, ½ cup at a time, into the butter mixture, stirring well after each addition.

4. Knead the dough a few times, form into a ball, and wrap in plastic wrap. Refrigerate at least 2 hours to chill.

5. When the dough is ready, preheat the oven to 375°F. Lightly grease a cookie sheet and set aside.*

6. Place ⅓ of the chilled dough at a time on a lightly floured surface, and roll it out to ½-inch thickness. With a 2-inch cookie cutter, cut shapes from the dough and place them on the cookie sheet. Bake for 8 to 10 minutes, or until golden brown.

* Instead of greasing a cookie sheet, you can cover it with parchment paper, which makes for quick and easy cleanup.

CHOCOLATE PECAN SANDIES

Yield: About 2 dozen

$\frac{3}{4}$ *cup unsalted (sweet) butter, softened*

1 ounce unsweetened baking chocolate, melted

$\frac{1}{4}$ *cup vegetable glycerine**

1 tablespoon water

1 tablespoon vanilla flavoring

$\frac{1}{4}$ *teaspoon white stevia powder*

2 cups all-purpose baking mix, sifted**

$\frac{1}{2}$ *cup finely ground pecans*

1 cup coarsely chopped pecans

* Derived from coconut oil, vegetable glycerine is a sweet-tasting thickener. It is available in most health food stores.

** Arrowhead Mills brand is recommended.

1. Place the butter in a large mixing bowl and whisk until light and fluffy. Add the chocolate, glycerine, water, vanilla, and stevia, and continue to whisk until smooth.

2. Using a wooden spoon, stir the finely ground pecans into the butter mixture, then add the baking mix, $\frac{1}{2}$ cup at a time, stirring well after each addition.

3. Add the coarsely chopped pecans to the dough. Knead the dough several times, form into a ball, and wrap in plastic wrap. Refrigerate 3 to 4 hours to chill.

4. When the dough is ready, preheat the oven to 375°F. Lightly grease a cookie sheet and set aside.*

5. Shape the dough into 2-inch balls and place them about 2 inches apart on an ungreased cookie sheet. Flatten the balls slightly with the bottom of a glass. Bake for 15 to 20 minutes, or until golden brown.

* Instead of greasing a cookie sheet, you can cover it with parchment paper, which makes for quick and easy cleanup.

CHOCOLATE TRUFFLES

Yield: About 40 truffles

8 ounces unsweetened chocolate
1¼ cups salted butter, softened
12 ounces heavy cream
1 tablespoon plus 1 teaspoon vanilla flavoring
1 tablespoon plus 1 teaspoon brandy
½ teaspoon white stevia powder (or to taste)

1. Break the chocolate into 1-inch pieces, then slowly melt it in a double boiler set over medium-low heat (the water should be simmering gently, not boiling).

2. Stir in the butter, 1 or 2 tablespoons at a time, until the mixture is smooth and glossy. Slowly stir in the cream and stevia.

3. Remove from the heat, then stir the vanilla and brandy flavorings into the chocolate until smooth and well combined. Pour into a shallow bowl and refrigerate about 45 minutes, or until firm.

4. Using a melon baller or teaspoon, scoop the chocolate into 1-inch balls and place them on a cookie sheet lined with waxed paper. Frequently dipping the melon baller in hot water will make forming the balls easier. Store uncovered in the refrigerator.

5. Before serving, let the truffles stand at room temperature about 30 minutes.

Variation

If desired, roll the just-formed truffles in crushed nuts, shredded coconut, unsweetened cocoa powder, or other decorative coatings.

DARK CHOCOLATE ALMOND CLUSTERS

Yield: About 20

8 ounces unsweetened chocolate
3 tablespoons grated orange rind
1 teaspoon orange flavoring
1 tablespoon rum flavoring
½ teaspoon white stevia powder (or to taste)
½ cup roasted, unsalted whole almonds

1. Break the chocolate into 1-inch pieces, then slowly melt it in a double boiler set over medium-low heat (the water should be simmering gently, not boiling).

2. Remove from the heat and slowly stir in the orange rind, orange flavoring, rum flavoring, and stevia, stirring until smooth and well combined.

3. Transfer the chocolate to a shallow bowl and refrigerate for 30 minutes, or until the chocolate begins to get firm. Stir in the almonds.

4. Drop heaping tablespoons of the mixture onto a cookie sheet lined with waxed paper. The clusters should be about 1-inch in diameter. Refrigerate 1 hour, or until the clusters are set.

Variation

Add any of your favorite chopped nuts or dried fruit to the clusters. Pecans, pistachios, peanuts, and raisins are popular choices.

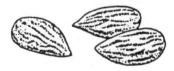

Fruit-'n-Nut Balls

Yield: 2 dozen

2 cups almonds
1 cup puffed brown rice
1 cup raisins
$\frac{1}{2}$ cup quinoa flakes
$\frac{1}{4}$ cup sesame seeds
$\frac{1}{4}$ cup almond butter
$\frac{1}{4}$ cup water
2 tablespoons liquid lecithin*
1 tablespoon vanilla flavoring
$\frac{1}{8}$ teaspoon white stevia powder

* Readily available in health food stores, lecithin is a flavorful, nutrient-rich binding agent that adds a creamy quality to products.

1. Place 1 cup of the almonds in a food processor and pulse to coarsely chop. And the remaining ingredients, continuing to pulse until the mixture is well combined. Transfer the mixture to a large mixing bowl.

2. Place the remaining cup of almonds in the food processor, and pulse to coarsely chop (these nuts should be slightly larger than the ones in the mixture).

3. Add the coarsely chopped nuts to the mixture, then return it all to the food processor. Continue to pulse until the mixture holds together to form a ball. (If the mixture does not hold together, add a teaspoon of water and continue to pulse.)

4. Shape the mixture into 2-inch balls and serve.

VANILLA ICE CREAM

If you have an ice cream maker, be sure to try this
stevia-sweetened recipe for classic vanilla ice cream.

Yield: About 1 quart

2 egg yolks
2 cups heavy cream
1 cup milk
2 teaspoons vanilla flavoring
$\frac{1}{2}$ teaspoon white stevia powder

1. In a blender, whip all of the ingredients very well, then refrigerate for about 45 to 60 minutes, or until chilled.

2. Pour the chilled mixture into an ice-cream maker and follow directions for freezing.

Variations

- Add fruit, carob or chocolate chips or nuts once mixture is semi-frozen, then complete freezing process.

- Garnish with Carob Fudge Sauce (page 105) and Sweet Whipped Cream (page 103).

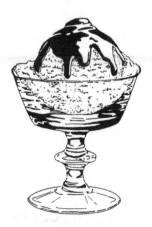

FRENCH CHOCOLATE ICE CREAM

This original recipe, for which you'll need an ice cream maker,
calls for 1 cup of sugar. By using a few drops of stevia liquid
concentrate, we were able to reduce the sugar ingredient to $\frac{1}{4}$ cup.

Yield: About 1 quart

1$\frac{1}{2}$ cups milk
3 egg yolks
$\frac{1}{4}$ cup sugar
8 drops stevia liquid concentrate
$\frac{1}{3}$ cup cocoa
2 cups heavy cream
1 to 3 teaspoons vanilla flavoring

1. Beat the milk and egg yolks together, then transfer the mixture to a 2-quart pot and place over medium heat. Stir in the sugar and cook, stirring constantly, for 4 to 5 minutes, or until the mixture is thick enough to coat the spoon. Remove from the heat.

2. Gently sprinkle the cocoa into the mixture, then return it to the heat, stirring until well blended.

3. Remove the mixture from the heat and let cool.

4. Stir the cream and vanilla into the cooled mixture. Refrigerate 45 to 60 minutes, or until well chilled.

5. Pour the chilled mixture into an ice-cream maker and follow directions for freezing.

BLUEBERRY ICE CREAM

A few simple ingredients and an ice cream maker
are all that you need for this luscious homemade treat.

Yield: About 1 quart

5 egg yolks
2 cups heavy cream
$\frac{1}{2}$ cup water
1 tablespoon vanilla flavoring
$\frac{1}{2}$ teaspoon white stevia powder
4 cups fresh blueberries

1. Blend all of the ingredients, except the blueberries, together in a large bowl, then refrigerate for 45 to 60 minutes, or until chilled.

2. Pour the chilled mixture into an ice-cream maker and follow directions for freezing.

3. When the mixture has started to become firm, fold in the blueberries, then continue to freeze.

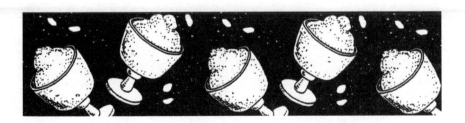

*L*USCIOUS *C*USTARDS, *P*UDDINGS, and *F*RUIT *T*REATS

BAKED CUSTARD (FLAN)

Yield: 4 cups

5 egg yolks
¼ teaspoon cinnamon
¼ to ½ teaspoon white stevia powder
4 cups milk
2 teaspoons vanilla flavoring
Pinch sea salt

1. Place oven rack in the lowest position, and preheat oven to 375°F.

2. Place the egg yolks, cinnamon, and stevia in a medium mixing bowl, and stir until well-combined (do not beat, as this will create foam). Set aside.

3. Place the milk in a 2-quart pot over medium-low heat and bring to a gentle simmer. Be careful not to scald the milk. Remove from the heat and cool slightly. Slowly stir the egg mixture into the cooled milk, stirring gently to minimize any foam. Add the vanilla and salt.

4. If the mixture has any lumps, pour it through a strainer into an 8-inch ovenproof baking dish or four individual ramekins. Skim any bubbles off the top.

5. Set the baking dish or ramekins in a deep, sturdy pan and place it the oven. Pour boiling water into the outer pan until it reaches halfway up the baking dish. Bake 35 to 40 minutes, or until the custard is firm and the top is golden brown. As the custard cooks, the water should be just simmering. (If the water boils, the custard will be grainy; if it is not hot enough, the custard will take hours to cook.)

6. Remove the pan from the oven, and carefully remove the custard from the water bath. Serve warm or chilled.

Variation

For a richer custard, replace half the milk with 2 cups half-n-half or heavy cream.

Vanilla Custard

Yield: 4 half-cup servings

2 eggs
2 teaspoons vanilla flavoring
¼ teaspoon white stevia powder
1 cup milk
1 cup heavy cream

1. Place the oven rack in the lowest position, and preheat the oven to 375°F.

2. Place the eggs, vanilla, and stevia in a medium mixing bowl, and stir until well-combined (do not beat, as this will create foam). Set aside.

3. Place the milk and cream in a 2-quart pot over medium-low heat and bring to a gentle simmer. Be careful not to scald. Remove from the heat and let cool slightly. Slowly stir the egg mixture into the cooled milk mixture, stirring gently to minimize any foam.

4. If the mixture has any lumps, pour it through a strainer into an 8-inch ovenproof baking dish or four individual ramekins. Skim any bubbles off the top.

5. Set the baking dish or ramekins in a deep, sturdy pan and place it the oven. Pour boiling water into the outer pan until it reaches halfway up the baking dish. Bake 35 to 40 minutes, or until the custard is firm and the top is golden brown. As the custard cooks, the water should be just simmering. (If the water boils, the custard will be grainy; if it is not hot enough, the custard will take hours to cook.)

6. Remove the pan from the oven, and carefully remove the custard from the water bath. Serve warm or cold, either plain or garnished with fruit.

BUTTERSCOTCH PUDDING

Yield: 4 cups

4 cups cooked, mashed butternut squash or yams
1 tablespoon butterscotch flavoring
$\frac{1}{2}$ teaspoon vanilla flavoring
$\frac{1}{8}$ teaspoon white stevia powder, or to taste

1. Preheat the oven to 350°F.
2. Place all of the ingredients in a blender or food processor and purée until very smooth.
3. Pour the mixture into an 8-inch baking dish or four individual ramekins.
4. Bake 25 to 30 minutes, or until the custard is firm and the top is golden brown.
5. Serve warm or chilled.

LEMON PUDDING

Yield: 6 cups

4 cups peeled, coarsely diced yellow squash
3 cups water
$\frac{1}{2}$ teaspoon white stevia powder
1 cup fresh lemon juice
2 tablespoons finely chopped lemon rind
4 heaping tablespoons agar flakes*

* Available in health food stores, agar—also known as kanten—is a natural gelling agent.

1. Place the squash, lemon juice, lemon rind, stevia, and 2 cups of water in a 2-quart pot. Place over medium heat, cover, and simmer about 10 minutes, or until the squash is soft.

2. Purée the mixture by passing it through a fine sieve. Set aside.

3. Place the remaining water and agar in a small saucepan. Simmer over very low heat, stirring frequently, until the agar is completely dissolved. Add the squash mixture and simmer another 5 minutes.

4. Pour into a bowl and refrigerate about 2 hours, or until gelled.

5. Once gelled, transfer the mixture to a blender and whip into a fluffy pudding.

6. Spoon into serving dishes and refrigerate another 30 minutes. Garnish with sliced fruit before serving.

CREAMY RICE PUDDING

Yield: 4 cups

3 cups water
$\frac{1}{2}$ teaspoon sea salt
1 cup basmati rice
1 cup heavy cream
$\frac{1}{2}$ cup raisins
$\frac{1}{2}$ cup shredded unsweetened coconut
1 teaspoon cinnamon
$\frac{1}{2}$ teaspoon nutmeg
$\frac{1}{4}$ teaspoon white stevia powder

1. Preheat the oven to 350°F.

2. Place 2 cups of the water in a 2-quart pot and bring to a boil over medium-high heat. Stir in the sea salt and rice, and bring to a second boil. Cover the pot, reduce the heat to low, and cook 30 minutes, or until the rice is tender.

3. Add the remaining water to the rice, along with the cream, raisins, coconut, cinnamon, nutmeg, and stevia. Mix well.

4. Spoon the mixture into an 8-inch ovenproof casserole dish and sprinkle with cinnamon. Bake for 25 to 30 minutes, or until the pudding is firm. Serve warm.

SWEET LEMONY TAPIOCA

Yield: 3 cups

2 ⅔ cups 2% low-fat milk, or unsweetened soy milk
6 3 tablespoons quick-cooking tapioca
2 teaspoons fresh grated lemon rind
1 tsp ¼ teaspoon white stevia powder
1 egg
1 teaspoon vanilla flavoring

1. Place the milk, tapioca, lemon rind, and stevia in a large mixing bowl and combine well. Beat the egg well and add it to the mixture. Let stand for 5 minutes.

2. Transfer the tapioca mixture to a 2-quart pot and place over medium-low heat. Bring to a gentle boil, stirring frequently to prevent the pudding from burning. When the mixture has reached a full boil, remove it from the heat. Add the vanilla and mix well.

3. Pour the mixture into 1-cup serving bowls. Cover the bowls with plastic wrap, and let the pudding cool at least 20 minutes before serving it warm. You can also refrigerate the pudding for several hours and serve chilled.

CHOCOLATE TAPIOCA

Yield: 3 cups

2 ⅔ cups 2% low-fat milk
3 tablespoons quick-cooking tapioca
1 tablespoon vanilla flavoring
½ teaspoon white stevia powder
1 egg
1 ounce unsweetened chocolate, crumbled

1. Place the milk, tapioca, vanilla, and stevia in a large mixing bowl and combine well. Beat the egg well and add it to the mixture. Let stand for 5 minutes.

2. In a double broiler set over medium-low heat, melt the chocolate until very smooth.

3. Transfer the tapioca mixture to a 2-quart pot and place over medium-low heat. Bring to a gentle boil, stirring frequently to prevent the pudding from burning. When the mixture has reached a full boil, remove it from the heat. Add the melted chocolate, stirring until well-combined.

4. Pour the mixture into 1-cup serving bowls, cover with plastic wrap, and refrigerate for several hours before serving.

SAVORY APPLESAUCE

Yield: 3 cups

1 teaspoon olive oil
2 medium Vidalia onions, finely diced
3 Rome apples, peeled and diced
1 tablespoon plus 1 teaspoon sea salt
½ cup organic, unrefined apple cider vinegar
¼ teaspoon cinnamon
⅛ teaspoon white stevia powder

1. Heat the oil in a 4-quart pot over medium heat. Add the onions and sauté for 3 to 4 minutes, or until translucent and lightly golden.

2. Add the apples and sea salt, reduce the heat to low, and simmer for 8 to 10 minutes, or until the apples are very soft.

3. Stir the apple cider vinegar, cinnamon, and stevia into the mixture, and continue to simmer another 5 minutes, stirring frequently.

4. Serve warm or cold.

CRANAPPLE RELISH WITH PECANS

Not only is this relish the perfect accompaniment for a traditional Thanksgiving dinner, it is also great mixed with kefir or organic fresh cream and enjoyed as a dessert. You can even add it to your favorite breakfast cereal.

Yield: 2 cups

1 tablespoon unsalted (sweet) butter
2 medium apples, peeled and finely diced
12-ounce package fresh cranberries
1 cup coarsely chopped pecans,
1 cup fresh orange juice
2 tablespoons fresh lemon juice
3 tablespoons finely chopped orange rind
1 tablespoon finely chopped lemon rind
1 tablespoon cornstarch
$\frac{1}{4}$ teaspoon cinnamon
$\frac{1}{4}$ teaspoon white stevia powder

1. Heat the butter in a large skillet over medium heat. Add the apples, cranberries, and pecans, and sauté for about 10 minutes, or until the apples and cranberries are soft.

2. Place the remaining ingredients in a small bowl and combine well. Add this mixture to the cranberry mixture and stir gently.

3. Simmer the ingredients and continue cooking until the mixture thickens slightly.

4. Transfer the relish to a bowl and refrigerate for several hours before serving.

BAKED APPLES

Yield: 6 apples

6 large Rome apples, peeled and cored
6 tablespoons unsalted (sweet) butter, softened
½ cup lemon juice
1 teaspoon grated lemon rind
½ teaspoon white stevia powder
1 teaspoon ground ginger
¼ teaspoon ground cloves
¼ teaspoon ground cardamom
¼ cup currants
¼ cup coarsely chopped almonds or pecans

1. Preheat the oven to 325°F.

2. Using a sharp knife, remove a ¼-inch piece from the top of each apple. Peel ¼-inch of skin from the top, and core each apple to within ½ inch of the bottom. Set aside.

3. Cream the butter with the lemon juice and lemon rind, then add the remaining ingredients. Spoon even amounts of this mixture into the cored apples.

4. Place the filled apples in a shallow baking pan, add a little water to cover the bottom, and bake for about 2 hours, or until tender. Serve hot, warm, or chilled.

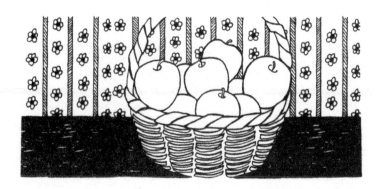

SWEET DRINKS ARE MADE OF THESE

HOMEMADE GINGER ALE

Yield: 8-ounce serving

3 ounces Ginger Syrup (below)
5 ounces sparkling mineral water
Ice cubes

1. Pour the syrup into a 10-ounce glass and add the ice cubes.

2. Slowly add the sparkling water. Stir and serve.

Making Homemade Ginger Syrup

With minimum effort, you can make this flavorful stevia-sweetened syrup to have on hand whenever you're in the mood for a refreshing glass of sparkling ginger ale. (See recipe above).

GINGER SYRUP

Yield: Approximately 4 cups

4 cups water
4- or 5-inch piece fresh ginger
$\frac{1}{2}$ teaspoon white stevia powder
2 tablespoons vanilla flavoring
1 tablespoon lemon extract

1. Peel and finely chop the ginger.

2. Bring the water to boil in small saucepan. Add the ginger and stevia, reduce the heat to low, and simmer gently for 8 to 10 minutes.

3. Strain the liquid into a heatproof container, and stir in the vanilla and lemon.

4. Covered and refrigerated, this syrup will keep for several days.

LEMONADE

Yield: Ten 8-ounce servings

2 cups fresh squeezed lemon juice
8 cups water
2 teaspoons stevia liquid concentrate
Ice cubes
Lemon slices for garnish

1. Combine all of the ingredients in a pitcher and stir until well-blended.

2. Pour into ice-filled 10-ounce glasses, garnish with lemon slices, and serve.

PIÑA COLADA SMOOTHIE

This smoothie is a nonalcoholic delight.

Yield: Two 8-ounce servings

1½ cups fresh pineapple juice
⅓ cup plain yogurt, or kefir
½ cup pineapple chunks
1 teaspoon coconut flavoring
⅛ teaspoon white stevia powder, or to taste

1. Place all of the ingredients in a blender and whip on high speed for 30 seconds.

2. Serve immediately.

CREAMY LIME DELIGHT

Yield: Two 8-ounce servings

$\frac{1}{2}$ cup freshly squeezed lime juice
1 cup plain yogurt, or kefir
$\frac{1}{4}$ teaspoon stevia liquid concentrate, or to taste
Pinch sea salt (optional)

1. Place all of the ingredients in a blender and whip on high speed for 30 seconds.

2. If smoothie is too thick, add a little filtered water to reach desired consistency. Serve immediately.

CREAMY CHERRY COOLER

Yield: Four 8-ounce servings

10-ounce package frozen cherries, slightly thawed*
2 cups plain yogurt, or kefir
12 drops stevia liquid concentrate, or to taste

* Organic Dark Sweet Cherries by Cascadian Farms is recommended.

1. Place all of the ingredients in a blender and whip on high speed for 30 seconds.

2. If smoothie is too thick, add a little filtered water to reach desired consistency. Serve immediately.

CREAMY ORANGE SURPRISE

Yield: Four 8-ounce servings

2 cups fresh squeezed orange juice
2 cups kefir,* or 1½ cups plain yogurt and ½ cup water
1 teaspoon vanilla powder or extract
10 drops stevia liquid concentrate, or to taste
Ice cubes

* A cultured, enzyme-rich beverage, kefir contains friendly bacteria and beneficial yeast that help balance the body's "inner ecosystem." It supplies complete protein, essential minerals, and valuable B vitamins. Kefir is sold in health food stores, or it can be made at home from a starter.

1. Combine all of the ingredients in a pitcher and stir until well blended.

2. Pour into ice-filled 10-ounce glasses and serve.

HOT COCOA

Yield: 8-ounce serving

8 ounces milk, or soy milk
2 teaspoons organic cocoa powder
⅛ teaspoon white stevia powder
½ teaspoon lecithin granules (optional)*

* This binding agent is readily available in health food stores.

1. Heat the milk in a small saucepan over medium-high heat until it just comes to a boil. Remove from the heat, add the remaining ingredients, and stir well.

2. Pour the hot cocoa into your favorite mug and top with Sweet Whipped Cream (page 103), if desired.

Variation

Instead of milk, try using flavored teas as the base for this hot cocoa. We have found Celestial Seasoning's Mint Magic, Vanilla Hazelnut, English Toffee, and Almond Sunset to be especially good, as well as Original Yogi Tea.

COFFEE LATTE

Yield: 8 cups

1$\frac{1}{4}$ cups regular grind espresso, or other dark roast coffee
1 cinnamon stick, broken into pieces
6 cups water
$\frac{1}{2}$ teaspoon white stevia powder, or to taste
2 $\frac{1}{2}$ cups skim milk, or 1 cup heavy cream and 1$\frac{1}{2}$ cups water
Ground cinnamon or nutmeg to taste

1. Brew the coffee and cinnamon in a drip or percolator coffee pot.

2. Add the stevia to the brewed coffee and mix well.

3. Heat the milk in a small saucepan over high heat until steam begins to rise (do not boil).

4. Pour half the heated milk into a blender and process at high speed about 15 seconds, or until it is foamy.

5. Pour the hot coffee into mugs or cups, then stir in the unblended milk. Spoon some of the foamed milk onto each serving, top with a sprinkling of cinnamon or nutmeg, and serve.

KOOL KEFIR SHAKE

This shake is the perfect morning breakfast drink.

Yield: 8-ounce serving

8 ounces plain kefir*
1 teaspoon flavoring: vanilla, blueberry, peach, banana, strawberry,
lemon, lime, orange, coconut, and almond are all good choices
2 to 4 drops stevia liquid concentrate
Ice cubes

* A cultured, enzyme-rich beverage, kefir contains friendly bacteria and beneficial yeast that help balance the body's "inner ecosystem." It supplies complete protein, essential minerals, and valuable B vitamins. Helios Nutrition, an organic kefir, is sold in health food stores, or it can be made at home from a starter.

1. Place all of the ingredients in a blender and process until well-blended.

2. Pour into an ice-filled 10-ounce glass and serve.

Variations

- To further enrich the nourishment of this drink, add any of the following:

  ❏ 1 teaspoon unrefined organic oil such as flaxseed, or pumpkin seed oil

  ❏ $1/_2$ teaspoon lecithin granules

  ❏ 1 teaspoon ground flaxseed

  ❏ 1 to 2 teaspoons probiotic powders—especially *L. acidophilus, B. bifidum,* and *L. bulgaricus.*

- Adding 2 to 3 ounces of thawed organic frozen fruit, such as strawberries, blueberries, or raspberries, makes this drink especially popular among children.

Resource List

In addition to the many health food stores located throughout the United States, the following companies provide stevia and many of the ingredients called for in this book.

Body Ecology
Atlanta, GA
1-800-511-2660
www.stevia.net

White stevia powder, stevia liquid concentrate, organic coconut oil, raw organic apple cider vinegar, xanthan gum, kefir starter culture, stevia recipes, and unrefined organic oils.

Now Natural Foods
Chicago, IL
1-800-999-8069

White stevia powder, stevia liquid concentrate, stevia tabletop packets.

Stevita Company, Inc.
7650 US Highway 287, #100
Arlington, TX 76001
1-817-483-0044
1-888-STEVITA
www.stevitastevia.com

White stevia powder with maltodextrin, stevia tabletop packets, liquid concentrate, dietary supplements, drink mixes, and pure stevia leaf powder.

Wisdom of the Ancients
Tempe, AZ
1-800-899-9908

White stevia powder, stevia liquid concentrate, stevia tea bags.

Bibliography

Abe, K., and M. Sonobe. *New Food Industry,* 19:1: 67, 1977.

Akashi, J., and S. Yokohama. "Safety of extract of dried Stevia leaves—results of toxicity tests." *Shokuhin Kogya,* 10B:34–43, 1975.

Alvarez, M., R.B. Bazzote, G.L. Godoy, et al. "Effect of aqueous extract of Stevia rebaudiana Bertone on biochemical parameters of normal adult persons." *Arq Biol Tech,* 24:178, 1981.

Aquino, R.P., I. Behar, A. Biondi, F. De Simone, and G. Scalesse. "Isolation of the principal sugars of Stevia rebaudiana." *Boll Soc Ital Biol Sper,* 61(9):1247–1252, 1985.

Bertoni, Moises. "Kaa he-he, its nature and its properties." *Paraguayan Scientific Annals,* 10 December, 1905.

Blackburn, G.L., B.S. Kanders, P.T. Lavin, S.D. Keller, and J. Whatley. "The effect of aspartame as part of a multidisciplinary weight-control program on short- and long-term control of body weight." *American Journal of Clinical Nutrition,* 65(2):409–418, 1997.

Boech, E.M.A., and G. Humboldt. "Cardio-circulatory effects of total water extract in normal persons and of stevioside in rats." *Ciencia e Cultura,* 32:208–210, 1981.

Brady, George. American Trade Commissioner's Memo for Latin American Division, August 31, 1921.

Bridel, M., and R. Lavielle. "Le principe a saveur sucree du Kaa'-he'-e (Stevia rebaudiana Bertoni)." *J Pharm Clin,* 14:99–154, 1931.

Brown, J.P. "A review of the genetic effects of naturally occurring flavonoids." *Mutation Res,* 75:243–277, 1980.

Crammer, B., and R. Ikan. "Progress in the chemistry and properties of rebaudioside." Greenby, T.H., editor. *Developments in Sweeteners.* London, Elsevier, vol 3:45–64, 1987.

Curi, R., M. Alvarez, R.B. Bazotte, L.M. Botion, J.L. Godoy, and A. Bracht. "Effect of Stevia rebaudiana on glucose tolerance in normal adult humans." *Brazilian Journal of Medicine & Biological Research,* 19(6):771–774, 1986.

D'Agostino, M., F. De Simone, C. Pizza, and R. Aquino. "Sterols in Stevia rebaudiana Bertoni." *Boll soc Ital Biol Sper,* 60(12):2237–2240, 1984.

Das, S., A.K. Das, R.A. Murphy, I.C. Punwani, M.P. Nasution, and A.D. Kinghorn. "Evaluation of the cariogenic potential of the intense natural sweeteners stevioside and rebaudioside A." *Caries Research,* 26(5):363–366, 1992.

Fletcher, Hewitt, Jr. "The sweet herb of Paraguay." *Chemurgic Digest,* 18, July/August, 1955.

Hubler, M.O., A. Bracht, and A.M. Kelmer-Bracht. "Influence of stevioside on hepatic glycogen levels in fasted rats." *Research Communications in Chemistry, Pathology, and Pharmacology,* 84:111–118, 1994.

Ishii, E.L., A.J. Schwab, and A. Bracht. "Inhibition of monosaccharide transport in the intact rat liver by stevioside." *Biochemical Pharmacology,* 36:9:1417–1433, 1987.

Ishii-Iwamoto E.L., and A. Bracht. "Stevioside is not metabolized in the isolated perfused rat liver." *Research Communications in Molecular Pathology and Pharmacology,* 87:167–175, 1995.

Isima, N., and O. Kakayama. "Sensory evaluation of stevioside as a sweetener." *National Food Research Institute,* 31:80–85, 1976.

Kelmer-Bracht, A., M. Alvarez, and A. Bracht. "Effects of Stevia rebaudiana natural products on rat liver mitochondria." *Biochemical Pharmacology,* 34(6):873–882, 1985.

Kinghorn, A.D., and D.D. Soejarto. "Current status of stevioside as a sweetening agent for human use." *Economic and Medicinal Plant Research,* London: Academic Press, Inc., 1985.

Kinghorn, A.D., D.D. Soejarto, N.P. Nanzakkara, C.M. Compadre, H.C. Makapugay, J.M. Hovanec-Brown, P.J. Medon, and S.K. Kamath. "A phytochemical screening procedure for sweet ent-kaurene glycosides in the genus Stevia." *Journal of Natural Products,* 47(3):439–444, 1984.

Klongpanichpak, S., P. Temcharoen, C. Toskulkao, S. Apibal, and T. Glinsukon. "Lack of mutagenicity of stevioside and steviol in *Salmonella typhimurium* TA 98 and TA 100." *Journal Medical Associations of Thailand,* Sep; 80, Suppl 1:S121–128, 1997.

Lee, C.K. "Carbohydrate sweeteners: structural requirements for taste." *World Review in Nutrition and Diet,* 33:142–197, 1979.

Matsui M., K. Matsui, Y. Kawasaki, Y. Oda, T. Noguchi, et al. "Evaluation of the genotoxicity of stevioside and steviol using six *in vitro* and one *in vivo* mutagenicity assays." *Mutagenesis,* 11:573–579, 1996.

Mauri, P., G. Catalano, C. Gardana, and P. Peitta. "Analysis of stevia glycosides by capillary electrophoresis." *Electrophoresis,* 17:367–371, 1996.

Melis, M.S. "Renal excretion of stevioside in rats." *Journal of Natural Products,* 55(5):688–690, 1992.

———. "Chronic administration of aqueous extract of Stevia rebaudiana in rats: renal effects." *Journal of Ethnopharmacology,* 47(3):129–134, 1995.

———. "A crude extract of Stevia rebaudiana increases the renal plasma flow of normal and hypertensive rats." *Brazilian Journal of Medicine & Biological Research,* 29(5):660–675, 1996.

Melis, M.S., and A.R. Sainati. "Effect of calcium and verapamil on renal function of rats during treatment with stevioside." *Journal of Ethnopharmacology,* 33(3):257–262, 1991.

Miyazaki, Y., H. Watanabe, and T. Watanabe. "Studies on the cultivation of Stevia rebaudiana Bertoni. Yield and stevioside content of 2-year-old plants." *Eisei Shikenjo Hokuku,* 96:86–89, 1978.

Mosettig E., and W.R. Nes. "Stevioside. The structure of the aglucon." *Journal of Organic Chemistry,* 20:884–899, 1955.

Nakayama, K., D. Kasahara, and F. Yamamoto. "Absorption, distribution, metabolism and excretion of stevioside in rats." *Journal of Food Hygiene Society Japan,* 27(1):1–8, 1986.

Nunes, P., and N.A. Pereira. "The effect of stevia rebaudiana on the fertility of experimental animals." *Revista Brasileira de Farmacia,* 69:46–50, 1988.

Oliveira-Filho, R.M., O.A. Uehara, C.A. Minetti, and L.B. Valle. "Chronic administration of aqueous extract of Stevia rebaudiana in rats: endocrine effects." *General Pharmacology,* 20(2):187–191, 1989.

Olney, J.W., N.B. Farber, E. Spitznagel, and L.N. Robins. "Increasing brain tumor rates: is there a link to aspartame?" *Journal of Neuropathology & Experimental Neurology,* 55(11):1115–1123, 1996.

Pezzuto, J.M., C.M. Compadre, S.M. Swanson, D. Nanayakkara, and A.D. Kinghorn. "Metabolically activated steviol, the aglycone of stevioside, is mutagenic." *Proceedings of the National Acadamy of Sciences,* 82(8):2478–2482, 1985.

Planas Mazzei, G., and J. Kuc. "Contraceptive properties of Stevia rebaudiana." *Science,* 162 (857):1007, Nov 29, 1968.

Schleicher, E., E. Wagner, and A. Nerlich. "Increased accumulation of the glycoxidation product N (epsilon)-(carboxymethyl) lysien in human tissues in diabetes and aging." *Journal of Clinical Investigations,* 99:457–468, 1997.

Schleicher, E., and O. Wieland. "Kinetic analysis of glycation as a tool for assessing the half-life of proteins." *Biochem Biophys Acta,* 884: 199–205, 1996.

Shibata, H., Y. Sawa, T. Oka, S. Sonoke, K.K. Kim, and S.M. Yoshioka. "Steviol and steviol-glycoside glucosyltransferase activities in Stevia rebaudiana Bertoni—purification and partial characterization." *Archives of Biochemistry and Biophysics,* 321(2):390–396, 1995.

Soejarto, D.D. "Potential sweetening agents of plant origin, field search for sweet-tasting Stevia species." *Economic Botany,* 77, 1983.

Soejarto, D.D., C.M. Compadre, et al. *Economic Botony,* 37:74, 1983.

Soejarto, D.D, A.D. Kinghorn, and N.R. Farnsworth. "Potential sweetening agents of plant origin. III. Organoleptic evaluation of Stevia leaf herbarium samples for sweetness." *Journal of Natural Products,* 45:590–599, 1982.

Suttajit, M., U. Vinitketkaumnuen, U. Meevatee, and D. Buddhasukh. "Mutagenicity and human chromosomal effect of stevioside, a sweetener from Stevia rebaudiana Bertoni." *Environmental Health Perspectives Supplement,* 101 (3):53–56, 1993.

Toskulkao, C., W. Deechakawan, et al. "Nephrotoxic effects of stevioside and steviol in rat renal cortical slices." Journal of Clinical Biochemistry and Nutrition, 16(2):123–131, 1994.

Toskulkao, C., and M. Sutheerawattananon. "Effects of stevioside, a natural sweetener, on intestinal glucose absorption in hamsters." *Nutrition Research*, 14(11):1711–1720, 1994.

Toyada, K., H. Matsui, T. Shoda, C. Uneyama, K. Takada, and M. Takahashi. "Assessment of the carcinogenicity of stevioside in F344 rats." *Food and Chemical Toxicology*, 35(6):597–603, 1997.

Uehara, O.A., V.H. Utino, et al. "Stevioside-androgen interactions." 7th Symposium Brazilian Medicinal Plants, Manaus, 1:74, 1982.

Von Schmelling, G.A., et al. "Stevia rebaudiana Bertoni: Evaluation of the hypoglycemic effect in alloxanized rabbits." *Ciencia e Cultura*, 29(5):599–601, 1977.

Wingard, P.E., J.P. Brown, et al. "Intestinal degradation and absorption of the glycosidic sweeteners stevioside and rebaudioside A." *Experientia*, 36, 519–520, 1980.

Wood, H.B., Jr., R. Allerton, H.W. Diehi, and H.G. Fletcher. "Stevioside. The structure of the glucose moieties." *Journal of Organic Chemistry*, 20:875–879, 1955.

Xili, L., B. Chengjiny, et al. "Chronic oral toxicity and carcinogenicity study of stevioside in rats." *Food Chemistry Toxicology*, 30:957–965, 1992.

Yamada, A., S. Ohgaki, T. Noda, and M. Shimizu. "Chronic toxicity study of dietary stevia extracts in F344 rats." *Journal of Food Hygiene Society Japan*, 26:169–183, 1985.

Yamamoto, N.S., A.M. Kelmer-Bracht, E.L. Ishii, F.S. Kemmelmeier, et al. "Effect of steviol and its structural analogues on glucose production and oxygen uptake in rat renal tubules." *Experientia*, 41(1):55–57, 1985.

Yodyingyaud, V., and S. Bunyawong. "Effect of stevioside on growth and reproduction." *Human Reproduction*, 6(1):158–165, 1991.

Index

T

V

W

Metric
Conversion Tables

Common Liquid Conversions

Measurement	=	Milliliters
$1/4$ teaspoon	=	1.25 milliliters
$1/2$ teaspoon	=	2.50 milliliters
$3/4$ teaspoon	=	3.75 milliliters
1 teaspoon	=	5.00 milliliters
$1^1/4$ teaspoons	=	6.25 milliliters
$1^1/2$ teaspoons	=	7.50 milliliters
$1^3/4$ teaspoons	=	8.75 milliliters
2 teaspoons	=	10.0 milliliters
1 tablespoon	=	15.0 milliliters
2 tablespoons	=	30.0 milliliters

Measurement	=	Liters
$1/4$ cup	=	0.06 liters
$1/2$ cup	=	0.12 liters
$3/4$ cup	=	0.18 liters
1 cup	=	0.24 liters
$1^1/4$ cups	=	0.30 liters
$1^1/2$ cups	=	0.36 liters
2 cups	=	0.48 liters
$2^1/2$ cups	=	0.60 liters
3 cups	=	0.72 liters
$3^1/2$ cups	=	0.84 liters
4 cups	=	0.96 liters
$4^1/2$ cups	=	1.08 liters
5 cups	=	1.20 liters
$5^1/2$ cups	=	1.32 liters

Converting Fahrenheit to Celsius

Fahrenheit	=	Celsius
200–205	=	95
220–225	=	105
245–250	=	120
275	=	135
300–305	=	150
325–330	=	165
345–350	=	175
370–375	=	190
400–405	=	205
425–430	=	220
445–450	=	230
470–475	=	245
500	=	260

Conversion Formulas

LIQUID		
When you know	Multiply by	To determine
teaspoons	5.0	milliliters
tablespoons	15.0	milliliters
fluid ounces	30.0	milliliters
cups	0.24	liters
pints	0.47	liters
quarts	0.95	liters

WEIGHT		
When you know	Multiply by	To determine
ounces	28.0	grams
pounds	0.45	kilograms